A BASIC GUIDE TO HERBS

USES, SIDE EFFECTS, INTERACTIONS AND OVERDOSE

Kay. A. Fox RN MSN CEN

ISBN-13:978-1-7369347-0-8

Cover design by: Art
Library of Congress Control Number: 2002092825
Printed in the United States of America

Dedication

This book is dedicated to my loving late Nana Kay. Nana, Thank you for inspiring me in all that I do, inspiring us all...You shared your talents and gifts with the world. This book has been reshaped to outlive and continue your powerful legacy, Thank you for teaching me to be a fighter and always go after my dreams! We miss you, & we will always love you!

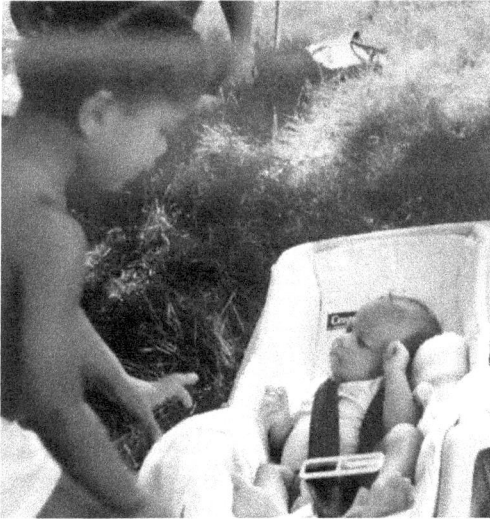

Introduction

This guide is for anyone interested in natural remedies, including health care providers. As we enter the new millennium, more people are turning to alternative, complementary, integrative forms of treatment.

Nature has shown us time and again, every action causes a reaction. You will find this guide lists the names of the herbs, their primary uses, potential side effects, interactions, and signs of overdose. As I found in my research, different sources listed different information on those issues. I have done my best to ferret out the most inclusive information available. The side effects, interactions and overdose sections may state "None reported". This only means that in my research these things were not reported. It would be reasonable to assume if there are side effects listed, an overdose would be an increase of those side effects. If you suspect an overdose, seek emergency treatment immediately.

The information presented here is a compilation of many sources and intended for educational purposes only. It is not intended as a substitute for the treatment, cure, diagnosis or mitigation of a disease or condition. Persons with potentially serious medical conditions should seek professional care.

Do not take any medications or herbals without first consulting with your physician. Any woman who plans to become pregnant, is pregnant or is breastfeeding must first talk with her doctor before taking any medication or natural remedy. Likewise, with children it is important to talk with their doctors before giving them over the counter or prescription any herbal, medications.

People with hormonal deficiencies or chronic problems with their gastrointestinal tract should not take many of these remedies and need to talk with their physicians. Some herbal remedies will interfere with the body's ability to absorb and use other medicines. The effectiveness of many natural remedies is just now being researched by science. As with many prescription medications, the manner in which these remedies effect their actions is unknown. Obviously, the only way to make your healthcare truly a team effort is to discuss your entire health history and give your physician the most complete information you have, including all the medications, herbals and over the-counter remedies you take.

The information contained within this guide is not to be considered a prescription therefore dosing information is not included. The purpose of this guide is simply to increase the readers' knowledge base so they may make intelligent, informed choices in their own care. For more detailed information, the reader may wish to examine the bibliography and continue with more research of their own
Use this guide in good health.

Table of Contents

THE HISTORY OF MEDICINE

2000 B.C. -Here, eat this root.
1000 A. D.-That root is heathen. Here, say this prayer.
1850 A.D. That prayer is superstition. Here, drink this potion.
1940 A.D. That potion is snake oil. Here, swallow this pill.
1985 A.D.-That pill is ineffective. "Here, take this antibiotic"
2000 A.D.- That antibiotic doesn't work anymore. "Here eat this root."

(Author unknown)

A CIRCLE COMPLETES AS WE RETURN TO NATURE FOR OUR HEALTH

A BASIC GUIDE TO HERBS-USES SIDE EFFECTS INTERACTIONS AND OVERDOSE

Aconite Monkshood, Blue Rocket, Aconitum nepellus: contains Aconine, Aconitine, Bezoylamine, Neopelline, Picratonitine

Uses. Decrease blood pressure. Decrease fever. Heartbeat irregularities. Increase sweating. Neuralgias. Nerve disorders. Stimulate the central nervous system and peripheral nerves.

Side Effects. Queasiness. Vomiting. Diarrhea. Urination. Interactions. Do not take this herb with any medications or herbals

Overdose. A dose of 5ml (about 1 teaspoon) can be lethal. Burning. Numbness of tongue and lips. Difficult swallowing. Irritability. Nausea. Restlessness. Speech difficulties. Blurred or double vision. Vomiting. Tingling of the mouth, fingers and toes, spreads over body and changes to flurry sensation. Body temperature falls. Irregular breathing. Death.

Adonis Vernalis False Hellebore, ox-eye, Phesant's Eye, Red Morocco, Rose-a-rubie, Sweet Vernal.

Uses. Cramps, Fever, Irregular heartbeat. Menstrual disorders. Weak heart. Water retention. Side effects. None reported.

Interactions. Digitalis-based drugs i.e. digoxin (Lanoxin). Do not take with potassium deficiency. Enhances action and side effects of: calcium supplements, diuretics (Hydrodiuril and Lasix), Laxatives, Quinidine (Quinaglute, Quinidex), Hydrocortisone. Prednisone.

Overdose. May be poisonous by vein.

Agave Century plant, Agave lecheguila: contains Diosgenin, Photosensitizing pigment, Steroidal chemicals, Vitamin C

Uses. Arthritis. Constipation. Disinfectant. Dysentery. Hair growth. Hormone replacement. Immunosuppressant. Nutrition.

Painful sprains. Stomachache. Syphilis (as disinfectant diuretic). Toothache I

Side Effects. Abortion or miscarriage (remote possibility). Disintegration of red blood cells. Irritate skin. Irritate lining of gastrointestinal tract. Small amounts depress central nervous system. Damaged cells. Change tissue permeability. Diarrhea. Increased sensitivity to sunlight. Jaundice (yellow eyes and skin). Nausea. Vomiting. Skin itching and rash. Unusual bleeding. May be caustic.

Interactions. Cortisone. ACTH. Testosterone. Androgenic steroids. May interfere with the absorption of vitamins, minerals and medications.

Overdose. None Reported.

Agrimonia eupatoria Church Steeples, Cocklebur, liverwort, Philanthropos, sticklewort

Uses. Bites, Bruises, Diarrhea, Heal wounds, Skin inflammation. Sore throat. Sprains. Stimulates bile flow. Warts.

Side Effects. Do not take if constipated.

Interactions. None

Overdose. None reported.

Adler Black Adler, Buckthorn, Rhamnus Frangula, Frangula: contains Anthraquinone glycosides, Emodin, Rhamnose

Uses. Cathartic. Constipation.

Side Effects: Irritate gastrointestinal tract. Severe abdominal cramps. Abdominal pain. Nausea. Vomiting. Loss of potassium. Irregular heartbeats. Kidney damage.

Interactions. None reported.

Overdose. Swelling. Accelerated bone deterioration. Irregular heartbeats. Kidney Damage.

Alfalfa Medicago sativa, Buffalo herb, Lucerne, Purple Medic: contains protein, saponin, flavones, isoflavones, sterols and coumarin derivatives.

Uses. Aids assimilation of nutrients. Anemia. Arthritis. Blood clotting. Cholesterol-lowering. Diabetes. Indigestion. Jaundice. Lactation. Loss of appetite. Menopause. Menstruation. Poultice for boils and inspect bites. Source of Vitamins A, B_1, B_6, C, E, K, calcium, potassium, iron, and zinc. Thyroid conditions. Water retention.

Side Effects. May cause systemic lupus erythematosus (SLE), a painful arthritis-like condition. Avoid sprouts if you have SLE (or similar condition). Damage red blood cells. Bleeding disorder. Anemia. If allergic to peas may also be allergic to Alfalfa.

Drug Interactions. Effects of blood thinners like warfarin sodium (Coumadin) or heparin maybe heightened. Do not take with Tegretol or Tetracycline.

Overdose. None reported

Allspice Jamaican Pepper, Clove Pepper, Pimenta dioica: Contains Acid-fixed oil. Eugenol, Resin, Tannic acid, Volatile Oils

Uses: Expel gas from intestines. Flavoring for food, toothpaste and other products. Relieve colic or griping. Relieve diarrhea. Relieve fatigue.

Side effects. Irritate mucous membrane. I.e. lining of gastrointestinal tract.

Interactions. May interfere with the absorption of vitamins, minerals or medications.

Overdose. Convulsions, Nausea. Vomiting.

Aloe, Aloe vera, Aloe barbadensis, Mediterranean Aloe, Barbados Aloe, Zanzibar Aloe, Aloe officinalis: contains Barbaloin (not present in Aloe vera) , Beta-barbaloin, Socaloin, Resin, Tannins, Anthraquinone glycosides splits to form aglycones

Uses. Abdominal pain, Antibacterial effect. Anti-inflammatory effects. Aphrodisiac. Burns. Cathartic laxative. Cause breasts to develop more quickly. Constipation. Colic. Diabetes. Digestive aid. Eye problems. Fleas. Frostbite. Hardening of the arteries. Headache. Herpes Simplex viruses. Indigestion. Intestinal infection. Kills pseudomonas aeruginosa (skin bacterium). Low back pain. Minor cuts. Poison oak. Suppressed menses. Stimulate wound healing. Sunburn. Tissue repair. Treat x-ray or radiation burns. Worms. Water retention.

Side effects. Allergy. Slow healing with severe burns and wounds. Aggravate constipation. Laxative dependency.

Interaction. Diuretics, i.e. Diuril and Lasix, steroid drugs i.e. prednisone, and licorice root. Increase effect of heart regulating drugs i.e. digitalis and digoxin (Lanoxin). May interfere with the absorption of vitamins, minerals or medications.

Overdose. Abdominal cramps. Bowel irritation. Diarrhea. High dose: Bloody diarrhea. Shock. Minor skin irritation (for external applications). Nausea. Red urine. Urinary frequency. Backache. pain on urination. Vomiting.

Alstonia. Bark Alstonia, constricta, Australian Fever Bush, Australia Quinine, Devil Tree, Dita Bark, Fever
Bark, Pali-mara: contains trace amounts of reserpine.

Uses. Anti-hypertensive effect. Combat spasms. Diarrhea. Fever. Malaria. Rheumatism. Uterine stimulant. Colitis. Nasal congestion. Fatigue. Impotence. Slowed reaction time. Use caution when handling machinery or driving.

Interactions. Do not combine with monoamine oxidase inhibitors (like Nardil or Parnate), alcohol, or barbiturates, digitalis-based drugs like Lanoxin, or quinidine products like Quinaglute and Quinidex, levodopa (Sinemet), or many common flu remedies and appetite suppressants.

Overdose. Depression. Heavy sedation. Severe drop in blood pressure.

Alum Root American Sanicle, Heuchera, contains Tannins

Uses. Douche. Heart disease. Prevent secretion of fluids. Prevent skin irritation. Shrink tissues.

Side effects. Burning. Indigestion. Edema (swelling of hands and feet). Jaundice (yellow eyes and skin). Nausea. Vomiting.

Interactions. May interfere with the absorption of vitamins, minerals or medications.

Overdose. None reported. It would be reasonable to assume an exaggeration of side effects; side effects outweigh any possible benefits. Not to be taken internally.

American Dogwood American Boxwood, Cornus florida: contains Betulic acid, Cornin

Uses. Infected skin rashes. Inspect bites. Kill bacteria in boils and carbuncles. Reduce fever.

Side effects. Irritate GI Tract. Cathartic. Uterine contractions.

Interactions. None report.

Overdose. Abortion. Dermatitis.

Angelica Angelica archangelica: contains Angelic acid, Resin, Volatile oils.

Uses. Anemia. Appetite loss. Combat digestive spasms Heart disease. High blood pressure Common cold. Gas. Improve bile flow. Increase perspiration. Indigestion

Remedy menstrual problems and symptoms of menopause Stimulate digestive juices. Thins mucus in lungs and bronchial tubes

Side effects. Sensitivity to sunlight. Not to be confused with Chinese Angelica or Dong Quai

Interactions. Avoid in diabetes or pregnancy.

Overdose. None reported.

Anise Pimpinella anisum: contains Anethole, Essential oils

Uses. Antibacterial. Appetite loss. Asthma. Bronchitis. Colds. Colic. Cough. Expectorant. Fever. Gas. Increase perspiration. Increase urine output. Infection. Kills lice. Mild muscle relaxant. Liver and gallbladder problems. Sore throat. Sweeten breath. Thins mucus from lungs and bronchial tubes. Upset stomach

Side effects. Do not take this herb if you are allergic to Anise or anethole. Seizures. Difficulty breathing. Hallucinations. Skin Nausea. Vomiting. irritation.

Interaction. None reported.

Overdose. None reported. It would be reasonable to assume an exaggeration of side effects

Arginine Natural sources: brown rice, carob, chocolate, nuts, oatmeal, popcorn, raisins, raw cereals, sesame, sunflower seeds, whole wheat products.

Uses. Build muscle, decrease obesity, ingredient of all proteins. Increase metabolism in fat cells, increase sperm count in males. Inhibit cancer, Speed wound healing, Stimulate human growth hormone. Stimulate immune system. Deficiencies are rare except in crash diets of only a few foods and are more common in total protein deficiency, rare in first world countries.

Side effects. Diarrhea. Nausea. Increase activity of herpes viruses. If allergic to any protein (eggs, milk or wheat) do not take.

Interactions. None reported.
Overdose. None reported.

Arnica

Uses. Boils. Bronchitis. Bruises. Chest pain. Common cold. Cough. Dislocations. Fatigue. Fever. Hardening of the arteries. Heart problems. Rheumatism. Severe uterine bleeding. Skin inflammation. Sore throat. Sprains. Tendency to infection. External applications. Insect bites. Inflamed veins. Antiseptic. Painkiller.

Side effects. Itching. Blisters. Ulcers. Dead skin. Interactions. Do not take with blood pressure medications.

Interactions. Do not take with blood pressure medication.

Overdose. Series heart problems. Severe irritation of the digestive tract. Vomiting. Diarrhea. Bleeding.

Artichoke Cynara scolymus

Use. Appetite loss. Digestive problems. Liver and gallbladder problems. Prevent recurrence of gallstones
Speed recovery.

Side effects. Stimulate flow of bile. Not to be taken with a bile duct blockage. Frequent contact may cause allergic reactions.

Interactions. Allergy to chrysanthemums may indicate a cross allergy to Artichoke.

Overdose. None reported.

Asafetida Devil 's Dung, Ferula, Assafoetida Ferula ' Foetida: contains Gum, Volatile oils, Resin has garlic like odor and bitter taste.

Uses Colic. Condiment. Constipation. Flavoring ingredient. Nerve disorders. Placebo effect. Thins mucus from the lungs and bronchial tubes. Worn around neck to repel evil.

Side effects. Irritate lining of gastrointestinal tract. Laxative.

Interactions. None reported.
Overdose. Diarrhea.

Asarabacca Asarum europaeum, Black Snakeroot, Canada Snakeroot, European Snakeroot, Coltsfoot,
Hazel wort, Heart Snakeroot, Indian Ginger, Southern Snakeroot, Vermont Snakeroot, Wild Ginger
Uses. Asthma. Bronchial spasms. Bronchitis. Chronic sneezing. Cough. Dehydration. Eye inflammations. Heart pain (angina). Liver disease. Local anesthetic. Loosens phlegm. Migraine. Nervous problems. Pneumonia. Promote menstruation. Trigger abortion. Vomiting.
Side effects. Do not use natural dried root. One compound of the root has caused liver cancer in mice.
Interactions. None reported.
Overdose. Burning of the tongue. Stomach pain. Diarrhea. Skin rashes. Partial paralysis.

Ash Fraxinus excelsior
Uses. Ant-inflammatory. Arthritis. Bladder disorders. Cold. Constipation. Fever. Gout. Pain-killer. Rheumatism. Tonic. Water retention.
Side effects. None reported.
Interactions. None reported.
Overdose. None reported.

Asian Ginseng Panax ginseng, Korean Ginseng, Chinese ginseng, Panax quinquefolius, Eleutherococcus senticosus
Uses. Agitation. Brighten eyes. Curb emotion. Enhance intellectual and physical performance. Enlighten the mind. Improve vitality. Increase energy. Increase wisdom. Longevity. Lower blood

sugar. Quiet the spirit. Repair the five viscera. Remove noxious influence. Stress. Support the immune function.

Side effects. Overstimulation. Hypertonia (increased muscle tone). Edema. Insomnia. Menstrual abnormalities. Breast tenderness.

Interactions. May decrease effectiveness of warfarin (decreased INR). Caffeine increases the risk of overstimulation, tachycardia or hypertension and gastrointestinal upset. Do not use if you have uncontrolled high blood pressure. Do not take with MAOIs. Do not take with steroids. Mania in patients on phenelzine. Do not take with diabetic medications. Do not take with lanoxin. Do not take with blood pressure medications.

Overdose. None reported. It would be reasonable to assume an exaggeration of side effects.

Asparagus Root Asparagus officinalis, Sparrow grass

Uses. Cough. Diarrhea. Diuretic. Kidney and bladder stones. Nervous problems. Urinary tract infections.

Side effects. Do not take with kidney disease or a weak heart. Drink plenty of liquids.

Interactions. None reported.

Overdose. None reported.

Astragalus Astragalus membranaceus, Milk Vetch, Huang qi, Yellow Leader: contains flavonoids, polysaccharides tri terpene glycosides, amino acids, trace minerals.

Uses. Abscesses. Acquired immune deficiency syndrome (AIDS). Alzheimer's disease. Asthma. Arthritis. Burns. Chronic colds and flu. Deficiency of chi. Diarrhea. Fatigue. Improves immune system. Loss of appetite.

Protect heart from the Nervousness. Night sweats.

Coxsackie B virus. Restore T-cell counts. Weakness. Side effects. Gas. Loose bowel movements. Not a cancer cure. Other plants in the Astragalus family are
toxic.

Interactions. None reported.
Overdose. None reported.

Balsam Picea excelsa, Fir, Spruce, Norway pine
Uses. Antibacterial. Bronchitis. Colds. Cough. Decongestant. Fever. Nerve pain. Rheumatism. Sore throat. Tendency to infection. External. Improve loca circulation.

Side effects. Bronchial asthma or spasm. Not for external use on acute skin disease, heart problems, a large skin injury, infectious disease, or unusually stiff muscles.

Interactions. None reported.
Overdose. None reported

Barberry Berberis vulgaris, Jaundice berry, mountain grape , pipperidge, sow berry: contains berbamine, berberine, berberrubine, columbamine , hydrastine, jatrorrhizine, oxyacanthine, palmatine

Uses. Aids iron absorption. Arthritis. Blood pressure. Bronchial constriction. Constipation. Diarrhea. Dilates blood vessels. Diuretic. Enlarge spleen. Fever. Gout. Hemorrhoids. Improve immune system. Increase the flow of bile. Indigestion. Kidney disease. Kill bacteria on skin. Liver and gallbladder problems. Low back pain. Malaria and parasite infections. Slows heart rate. Tendency to infection. Urinary tract infections. Tuberculosis. Vitamin C.

Side effects. None reported. Use is discouraged.
Interactions. None reported. May interfere with the absorption of vitamins, minerals or medications.

Overdose. Depress breathing. Mild stupor. Nosebleeds. **Vomiting.** Diarrhea. Kidney irritation.

Barley Hordeum distychum, Pearl barley, pot barley, scotch barley: contains ash, cellulose, hordenine, invert sugar lignin, malt, nitrogen, pectin, pentosan, protein, starch, sucrose
    Uses. Abrasions. Diarrhea. Indigestion. Inflammation of stomach and bowels. Nutrition.
    Side effects. Avoid if allergic or sensitive to barley or gluten.
    Interactions. None reported.
    Overdose. If infected with fungus can cause poisoning.

Basil Ocimum basilicum, St. Joseph wort: member of the mint family contains linalool, methyl chavicol and eugenol
    Uses. Appetite stimulant. Bad breath. Circulation. Clouded vision. Colds. Depression. Diuretic. Earache. Fever. Gas. Indigestion. Kidney disease. Rheumatism. Stomach cramps. External. Bruises. Inflammation. Ringworm. Wounds.
    Side effects. None reported.
    Interactions. None reported.
    Overdose. None reported.

Bayberry Myrica cerifera, candleberry, tallow shrub ' wax myrtle, waxberry: contains gallic acid, mycricic acid, palmitinin, myricinic acid related to saponin' resin, tannic acid
    Uses. Astringent. Bronchitis. Common cold. Cough. Diarrhea. Induces perspiration. Insomnia. Jaundice. Liver conditions. Prevents secretion of fluids. Stimulant. External. Gums. Skin problems. Ulcers
    Side effects. Vomiting. Cancer in lab animals Interactions. None reported.

Overdose. None reported. It would be reasonable to assume an exaggeration of side effects.

Beans Phaseolus vulagris
Uses. Diabetes. Diuretic. Heart conditions. Kidney and bladder stones. Urinary tract infections.
Side effects. Stomach problems.
Interactions. None reported. May interfere with the absorption of vitamins, minerals or medications.
Overdose. Vomiting. Diarrhea. Stomach pain.

Bearberry Arctostaphylos, uva-uris, barberry, bearsgrape, kinnickinick , mealberry, mountain box, mountain cranberry, sandberry: contains arbutin, ericolin, galic acid, hydroquinolone, malic acid, quercetin, tannins, ursolic acid, volatile oils.
Uses. Breathing problems. Increase amount of urine produced. Nausea. Prevent secretion of fluids. Ringing in ears. Sedative. Shrink urinary tissues. Urinary tract infections. Urinary pain.
Side effects. Bad taste. Inflame the lining of the bladder and urinary tract.
Liver damage Nausea. Vomiting. Turns urine green.
Interactions. Acid urine decreases effectiveness
Overdose. None reported.

Bee balm Monarda
Uses. Acne. Alzheimer's disease. Cough. Diuretic.
Flu. Gas. Headache. Heart trouble. Hysteria.
Insect repellent. Insomnia. Measles. Parasites. Regulate menses. Sore throat. Stomachache.
Side effects. None reported.

Interactions. None reported.
Overdose. None reported.

Bee pollen contains some vitamins, minerals and amino acids
Uses. Anti-aging agent. Arthritis. Decrease allergy symptoms. Energize body. Heart disease. Improve immunity. Inhibit cancer. Prostate problems. Regulate bowels. Renew skin. Stress. Weight control.
Side effects. Itching, pain at injection site and swelling. Allergic reactions in people sensitive to pollens.
Interactions. None reported.
Overdose Anaphylaxis. Immediate severe itching. Paleness. Low blood pressure. Loss of consciousness. Coma.

Belladonna Atropa Belladonna, black cherry, deadly nightshade
Uses. Asthma. Bronchial asthma. Bronchitis. Bulging eyeballs from an overactive thyroid. Drying effect. Excessive perspiration. Intestinal and digestive pain and spasms. Irregular heartbeat. Liver and gallbladder Problems. Muscular pain. Nerve pain. Scarlet fever. Spasms of the heart muscle. Weak heart. External. Gout. Ulcers. Active ingredient in drugs like Donnatal and Levsin.

Side effects. Interferes with a chemical of nervous system, acetylcholine. Over-excitement. Hallucinations. Muscular tremor or rigidity.
Interactions. Increase side effects of Amatadine (Symmetrel) Quinidine (Quinaglute, Quinidex), Tricyclic antidepressant medications such as Elavil, Pamelor and Tofranil.
Overdose. Red skin. Dry mouth. Abnormal heartbeat. Prolonged or excessive pupil dilation. reduced Inability to focus.

Overheating due to perspiration. Difficult urination. Severe or persistent constipation. Over-excitement. Restlessness. Compulsion to talk. Hallucinations. Delirium. Manic attacks followed by exhaustion and sleep. Asphyxiation.

Bilberry Vaccinium myrtillus, Dyeberry, Huckleberry, Trackleberry, Whortleberry, Wineberry: related to blueberries, contains Anthocyanosises, a bioflavonoid complex, are reported to be potent antioxidants. Catechins, invertase, flavone glycosides (particularly of malvidin, cyanidin and delphinidin) and anthocyanosises

Uses. Antioxidant. Astringent. Break down plaque on artery walls. Connective tissue. Diabetes. Diarrhea. Gargle. Gout. Kidney stones. Improve capillary and venous blood flow. Improve health of the circulatory system. Night vision. Reduce platelet aggregation. Rheumatism. Scurvy. Skin inflammation. Sore throat. Stimulate gastric mucus. Stimulate new capillary formation. Stomach upsets. Strengthening capillary walls. Urinary tract infections. Vasodilator.

Side effects. Stomach upset. Do not take if diabetic • Increases tendency to bleed.

Interactions. None reported. Do not take with blood thinners or aspirin.

Overdose. Anemia. Malnutrition. Jaundice (yellowing of the skin and whites of the eyes).

Birch Betula alba, Betula Lenta, Silver Birch, White Birch: contains Betulin in bark, Methyl Salicylate similar to aspirin in bark, resin in shoots and leaves, tar creosol, phenol, creosote, guaicol in bark

Uses. Arthritis. Congestive heart failure. Decrease soft tissue inflammation. Diuretic. Fever. Kidney and bladder stones. Prevent secretion of fluids. Rheumatism. Urinary tract infections. External. Counter-irritation when applied to skin over an inflamed or irritated joint.

Side effects. May have cancer-causing compounds. Do not use if water retention is from reduced heart or kidney function. Drink extra fluid.

Interactions. None reported.

Overdose. None reported.

Birthroot Bethroot, Trillium erectum, Trillium pendulum: contains resin, saponin, starch, tannins, volatile oils

Uses. Aphrodisiac. Astringent. Bleeding after childbirth. Gastrointestinal upsets. Heartbeat irregularities. Menstrual irregularity or increased menstrual frequency. Prevent secretion of fluids. Skin infections. Shrink tissues. Thins mucus from lungs and bronchial tubes.

Side effects. Irritate mucous membranes.

Interactions. None reported.

Overdose. None reported.

Bistort Polygonum bistort, Adderwort, Dragonwort, Easter Giant, Oderwort, Osterick, Patience Dock, Red Legs, Snakeweed, Sweet Dock, Twice Writhen: contains tannins

Uses. Uses. Can be roasted and eaten. Diarrhea. Epilepsy. Fever. Gargle. Swollen glands. Tetanus. External. Burns. Cavities in teeth. Prevent secretion of fluids. Shrink tissues. Wounds. Unusual bleeding.

Side effects. Precipitates proteins. Vomiting.

Interactions. None reported.

Overdose. Dangers outweigh benefits. Bleeding from stomach. Vomiting bright-red blood or coffee ground appearing

material. Kidney damage. Blood in urine. Decreased urine flow.
Swelling of hands and feet.
Nausea.

Bitter Lettuce Lactuca virosa, Lactuca sa tiva, Lactuca scariola.
Latex from stem of flower stalks: contains caoutchouc, hyoscyamine,
lactucerol, lactucin, latucic acid, mannite, nitrates, volatile oils.
Uses. Angina. Anxiety. Cough. Depress central nervous
system. Nervous disorders. Sedative.
Side effects. Causes a "high" when smoked. Breathing
difficulties.
Interactions. None reported.
Overdose. Dangers outweigh benefits.

Bitter melon Mornordica charantia: contains steroidal
saponins, charantin, insulin-like peptides and alkaloids
Uses. Cancer. Diabetes.
Infections. Inhibit AIDS virus in test tubes. Psoriasis.
Side effects. Abdominal pain. Diarrhea. Cause or lower low
blood sugar.
Interactions. Increase effectiveness of hypoglycemic drugs or
insulin.
Overdose. None reported.

Bitter Orange Bitter Orange Bigarade Orange, Neroli
Uses. Appetite loss. Chest pain. Flavoring in liqueur
Curacao. Digestive tract spasms. Gastric complaints
Gout. Headache. Indigestion. Insomnia. Nervousness. Sore throat.
Vomiting.Pain.
Side effects. Skin irritation with redness, and blisters. Increase
sensitivity to sunlight.

Interactions. None reported.
Overdose. None reported.

Bitter Root Wild Ipecac, Spreading
Dogbane, Rheumatism Weed, Apocynum androsaemifolium:
apocynein, apocynin, cymarin, saponin
Uses. Bile flow. Congestive heart failure. Diuretic. Gallstones.
Palpitations. Restore normal
tone to tissues. Slow heartbeat. Stimulate appetite. Side effects.
Vomiting.
Interactions. Must take increased potassium.
Overdose. Precipitous blood pressure drop. Faintness. Cold
sweat. Paleness. Rapid pulse. Gastritis. Vomiting.

Bittersweet European bittersweet, bitter nightshade,
felonwood, solanum dulcamara : contains dulcamarin saponin,
solanidine, solanine
Uses Aphrodisiac. Arthritis. Depress central nervous system.
Eczema. Lymphatic medicine. Ovaries. Pain. Pancreas. Skin diseases.
Thyroid.
Side effects. Burning throat. Coma. Dilated pupils. Dizziness
Headache. Muscle weakness. Nausea. Slow pulse, Vomiting.
Interaction. None reported.
Overdose. Depress nervous system. Drowsiness. Berries are
poisonous. Dangers outweigh benefits.

Blackberry Rubus fruticosus, Bramble , Dewberry, Goutberry,
Thimbleberry, Tanin
Uses. Boils. Diarrhea. Diuretic. Protection from "evil runes".
Rheumatism. Sore throat. Snake bites.
Side effects. None reported.

Interactions. None reported.
Overdose. None reported.

Black Mustard Brassica nigra, brown mustard, red mustard: contains allylisothio cyanate
   Uses. Epilepsy. Hay fever. Runny nose. Snake bites. Sore throat. Warm and quicken spirits. External. Bronchial pneumonia. Pleurisy.
   Side effects. Blisters on skin. Irritate mucous membranes. Stomach problems. Kidney irritation. Inhaling vapors. Asthma attacks. Cough. Eye irritation. Sneezing.
   Interactions. None reported.
   Overdose. Vomiting. Stomach pain. Diarrhea. Sleepiness. Heart problems. Breathing difficulties. Coma. Death.

Black Root Leptandra virginica, Beaumont root, Bovman's root, Culver' s root, Oxadoddy, Physic Root,
Tall speedwell, Tall Veronica, Whorlywort
   Uses. Constipation. Gas. Liver and gall bladder problems. Promote perspiration. Vomiting.
   Side effects. None reported.
   Interactions. None reported.
   Overdose. None reported.

Blackthorn Prunus spinosa, Sloe, Wild plum
   Uses Astringent. Bloating. Cramps. Diarrhea. Indigestion. Inflammations of mouth. Laxative. Nerve pain. Nervous headaches. Sore throat. Urinary problems. Weak heart. Ingredient in sloe gin.
   Side effects. None reported.
   Interactions. None reported.
   Overdose. None reported.

Black Walnut Juglans nigra, Butternut, Lemon Walnut, Oilnut, White Walnut: contains Ellagic acid, Juglone, Nucin

Uses. Anti-tumor activity. Astringent. Fights bacteria and worms. Fungal infections of skin. Headache. Hemorrhoids. Hepatitis. Laxative. Liver and gallbladder problems. Prevent secretion of fluids. Skin condition. Brown dye for hair and clothes.

Side effects. None reported.

Interactions. None reported.

Overdose. Nausea. Upper abdominal pain

Bladderwrack Fucus vesiculosus, Black- tang, Cutweed, Kelpware, Quercus marina, Seawrack: contains Alginic acid Bromine Iodine, Fucodin, Laminarin

Uses. Bulk laxative. Excess weight. Hardening of arteries. High cholesterol. Indigestion. Insufficient thyroid. Kill intestinal parasites.

Side effects. Iodide can cause or worsen an overactive thyroid. Allergic reactions. May contain heavy metal pollution.

Interactions. Thyroid medication.

Overdose. Agitation. Fatigue. Increased appetite. Increased sweating. Insomnia.

Blessed thistle Cnicus benedictus, Cardin, Holy Thistle, Spotted Thistle, St. Benedict Thistle: contains sesqui terpene lactones such as cnicin.

Uses. Anti-inflammatory. Appetite loss. Constipation. Digestive problems. Gas. Headaches. Improve the flow of milk. Increases stomach secretion. Liver and gallbladder disease. Migraines. Stomach upset.

Side effects. Use cautiously if allergic to plants in the daisy family. Sensitivity to mugwort and cornflower.
Interactions. None reported.
Overdose. Handling can cause toxic effects on skin.

Bloodroot Sanguinaria canadensis, Coon Root, Indian Paint, Snakebite, Sweet Slumber, Tetterwort
Uses. Cough medicine. Dental plaque. Gingivitis. Gum disease
Side effects. Vomiting.
Interactions. None reported.
Overdose. Vomiting. Diarrhea. Cramping. Collapse. Poisoning.

Blueberry Vaccinum spp: contains Fatty acids, Hydroquinone, Loeanolic acid, Neomyrtillin, Tannins, Ursolic acid
Uses. Decrease blood sugar. Diarrhea. Diuretic. Gastroenteritis. Scurvy.
Side effects. None reported. May change color of stool.
Interactions. None reported.
Overdose. None reported.

Blue Mallow Malva Sylvestris, Cheeseflower, Mallow, Mauls
Uses. Bladder problems. Bronchitis. Coats irritate membranes. Cough. Stomach inflammation. Wounds
Side effects. None reported.
Interactions. None reported. May interfere with absorption of vitamins, minerals or medications.
Overdose. None reported.

Bog Bean Menyanthes trifoliata, Bean Trefoil, Bog Myrtle, Buck Bean, Marsh Clover, Moonflower, Water
Shamrock, Water Trefoil

Uses. Appetite loss. Diabetes. Headache. Indigestion. Urinary problems.
Side effects. Diarrhea or intestinal inflammation (colitis)
Interactions. None reported.
Overdose. None reported.

Boneset Eupatorium perfoliatum, E. rugosum, Agueweed, Crosswort, Feverwort, Indian Sage, Teasel, Thoroughwort: contains Eupatroin Resin, Sugar, Tremetrol, Volatile oils, Wax
Uses. Decrease blood sugar. Digestive problems. Fever. Flu. Improve immune system. Liver disorders. Malaria. Promote perspiration. Soothe inflammation.
Side effects. Allergic reaction. Excessive sweating. Diarrhea. Vomiting. Irritates gastrointestinal tract. Can cause a set of symptoms trembling, vomiting and severe abdominal pain, caused by products from cattle poisoned by eating boneset.
Interactions. None reported.
Overdose Coma. Drooling. Muscle trembling. Breathing difficulties. Nausea. Stiffness. Vomiting. Weakness.

Borage Borago officinal is
Uses. Coughs. Diuretic. Eczema. Expectorant. Fever. Irritable bowel syndrome. Menstrual regulation. Promote lactation. Rheumatism. Stimulates adrenals.
Side effects. None reported.
Interactions. None reported.
Overdose. None reported.

Boswellia Boswellia serrata, Salad guggal, produces a Gummy oleoresin resin, referred to as guggal , gum oleoresin: contains essential oils, gum and terpenoids, boswellic acids

Uses. Anti-inflammatory. Arthritis. Bursitis. Diarrhea. Dysentery. Lung disease. Osteoarthritis. Rheumatoid arthritis. Ringworm.

Side effects. Diarrhea. Skin rash. Nausea.
Interactions. None reported.

Overdose. None reported. It would be reasonable to assume an exaggeration of side effects.

Brewer's Yeast Saccharomyces cerevisiae
Uses. Acne. Appetite loss. Boils. Bronchitis. Colds. Cough. Diabetes. Eczema. High cholesterol. Indigestion. Infection. Kill bacteria. Promote production of certain white blood cells. Sore throat. Source of B vitamins, proteins and minerals.

Side effects. Diarrhea. Migraine headaches. Nausea.
Interactions. Increase in blood pressure when combined with a monoamine oxidase inhibitor (like antidepressants Nardil and Parnate) and Eldepryl (for Parkinson's).

Overdose. None reported. It would be reasonable to assume an exaggeration of side effects.

Broom Cytisus scoparius, Green Broom, Irish Broom Irish Tops, Scoparium, Scotch Broom
Uses. Arteriosclerosis. Blood purifier. Chest pain '
Enlarged spleen. Gall and kidney stones. Gout. Heald menstruation. Hemophilia. Hemorrhage after delivery •
Irregular heartbeat. Liver disorders. Low pressure. Respiratory conditions. Rheumatism. Sciatica. snake bites. Tense or stiff muscles. Water retention. Weak heart.

Side effects. None reported.

Interactions. Increase in blood pressure with monoamine oxidase inhibitors i.e. antidepressants Nardil and Parnate and Eldepryl (Parkinson' s medication).
Overdose. Dizziness. Headache. Palpitations. prickling in the extremities. Weakness in the legs. Sweating. Sleepiness. Pupil dilation. Eye problems. Asphyxiation.

Buchu Barosma betulina, Honey Buchu, Short-leaved Mountain Buchu: contains Diasmin, Hesperidin, I-enthone, Mucilage, Resin, Volatile Oils
Uses. Bladder irritation. Diuretic. Gas. Gout. Increases perspiration. Kidney stones. Prostate conditions. Rheumatism. Stimulates central nervous system. Urethral irritation. Urinary tract infections. Side effects. Skin irritation. Nausea. Vomiting.
Interactions. None reported.
Overdose. None reported. It would be reasonable to assume an exaggeration of side effects.

Buckthorn Rhamnus carthartica, Hartshorn, Highwaythorn, Rams thorn, Waythorn: contains Anthra quinone Emodin
Uses. Anal fissures. Constipation. Diuretic. Hemorrhoids. Recent rectal surgery. Softens stool.
Side effects. Do not take with; intestinal obstruction, acute inflammatory intestinal disorder, Ulcerative colitis, appendicitis or any abdominal pain. May cause potassium deficiency, intestinal dysfunction, heart problems, kidney disease, swelling and bone problems.
Interactions. Diuretics such as Diuril and Lasix. Steroid drugs like prednisone. Licorice root. Drugs like digitalis and digoxin (Lanoxin). Medicines for control of heartbeat. Do not take with these medicines.

Overdose. Excessive doses can be poisonous. Irritates gastrointestinal tract. Causes watery, explosive bowel movements. Kidney damage. Blood in urine. Decreased urine flow. Swelling of hands and feet. Nausea. Vomiting.

Bugleweed Lycopus virginicus, Gypsywort, Sweet Bugle, Water Bugle, Virginia Water Horehound
Uses. Inhibits action of thyroid hormones and reproductive hormones. Insomnia. Nervousness. Painful breasts. Premenstrual syndrome (PMS). Reduces levels of prolactin. Tension.
Side effects. Not for use with thyroid insufficiency. Do not take if having tests involving radioactive isotopes.
Interactions Do not take with thyroid medications. Do not take with heart medications. Do not take with diuretics. Do not take with antacids.
Overdose. Enlargement of the thyroid gland. Do not stop taking suddenly.

Bupleurm Bupleurum chinense, Hare's Ear, Thorowax Root
Uses. Bloated stomach. Chills. Fever. Flu. Indigestion. Irritability. Malaria. Menstrual problems • Nausea. Pressure in the chest. Tuberculosis. uterine prolapse. Vertigo.
Side effects. Nausea.
Interactions. None reported.
Overdose. None reported.

Burdock Arctium lappa, Bardane, Beggar's Buttons, Cocklebur, Edible Burdock, Great Burdock, Hareburr
Lappa: contains inulin, mucilage Arctiin, Inulin, Tannins, Volatile oils

Uses. Antimicrobial activity. Blood purifier. Cancer. Colds. Coughs. Deep skin infections. Digestion. Diuretic. Eczema. Fever. Gastrointestinal upset. Gout. Lower blood sugar. Measles. Painful joints. Psoriasis. Rheumatism. Skin disorders. Sore throats. Stimulates body's defenses. Tonsillitis. Ulcers. Urinary tract infections. Sore throats.

Side effects. None reported.

Interactions. Interferes with diabetic medicines.

Overdose. May be contaminated by atropine- like chemicals that can be poisonous. Dilated pupils. Dry mouth. Hallucinations.

Butcher's broom Ruscus aculeatus, Jew's Myrtle, Knee Holly, Kneeholm, Pettigree, Sweet Broom is in The lily family and similar to asparagus contains: steroidal molecules, ruscogenin, neoruscogenin

Uses. Anti-inflammatory. Diuretic. Hemorrhoids. Itching and burning of hemorrhoids. Laxative. Lower leg cramps, pain, itching, and swelling. Urinary problems. Vein problems.

Side effects. None reported.

 Interactions. None reported. Overdose. Stomach problems.

Cabbage Brassica oleracea var. capitata

Uses. Abdominal disorders. Bronchitis. Cough. Diarrhea. Poor digestion. Protect stomach from gastric acids Rheumatism. Skin diseases. Snake bite. Stomachache. Ulcers. Worms.

Side effects. None reported.

Interactions. None reported

Overdose. None reported

Cajuput Oil Melaleuca Leucadendron, Paper bark Tree, White wood

Uses. External. Antiseptic. Bruises. Low back pain. Muscle tension. Pulled muscles or ligaments. Rheumatism. Sciatica. Slipped disk. Sprains.

Side effects. Skin inflammation. Inhaled may interfere with breathing or cause throat spasms.

Interactions. None reported.

Overdose. None reported. It would be reasonable to assume an exaggeration of side effects.

Calamus Acorus calamus, Acore, Rat Root, Sweet Root, Sweet Flag, Sweet Cane, Cinnamon Sedge, Sweet Sedge,
Sweet Myrtle, Flagroot: contains Asarone, Beta-asarone, Camphene, Caryophyllene, Eugenol, Pinene, Volatile oils

Uses. Aphrodisiac. Appetite improvement. Asthma. Bronchitis. Chest pain (angina). Convulsions. Coughs. Dyspepsia. Epi lepsy. Fever Gas. Gum disease.
Indigestion. Insanity. Intestinal parasites. Hysteria.
Nervousness. Spasms. External. Circulation. Rheumatism.

Side effects. Depress central nervous system. Hallucinations.

Interactions. None reported.

Overdose. None reported. Avoid long-term use. The FDA has banned all varieties of this plant for human use

Calendula Calendula officinalis, Marigold: contains flavonoids, tri terpene, saponins, carotenoids.

Uses. Bile production. Regulates menstruation. Stomach inflammation. Stomach ulcers. External Antifungal. Anti-inflammatory. Antiseptic. Astringent. Eczema. Skin diseases. Skin ulcers. Wound healing. Sterile tea applied for conjunctivitis.

Side effects. None reported.

Interactions. None reported.
Overdose. Allergic reaction.

Carob Ceratonia siliqua, St. John's bread: contains large carbohydrates (sugars) and tannins.
Uses. Diarrhea. Gastric reflux. Inactivate toxins. Inhibit growth of bacteria.
Side effects. None reported.
Interactions. None reported.
Overdose. Allergic reactions.

California Poppy Eschscholtzia californica, Africa Pepper, American Pepper, Red Pepper, Spanish Pepper: contains Copt i sine, Sanguinarine
Uses. Aches. Agitation. Anxiety. Bedwetting. Bladder and liver diseases. Chronic fatigue. Depresses central nervous system. Depression. Feeble narcotic actions. Increases perspiration. Insomnia. Migraine-type headaches. Mood swings. Nervous disorders. Neuroses. Weather sensitivity.
Side effects. None reported.
Interactions. Do not take with barbiturates, valium-type medications or alcohol.
Overdose. None reported.

Camphor Cinnamomum camphora, Cemphire
Uses. Asthma. Blood pressure. Bronchial spasms. Bronchitis Circulation. Cough. Improves breathing. Indigestion. Inflammation. Irregular heartbeat. Muscle pain. Rheumatism. Weak heart. External. Stimulates circulation. Active ingredient in Vicks VapoRub and Mentholatum ointment. Inhaled. Reduce bronchial secretions. Moth-repellent.

Side effects. Skin irritation. Eczema.
Interactions. None reported.
Overdose. Can be fatal. Intoxication. Delirium. Spasms. Breathing difficulties.

Capsicum Capsicum frutescens, capsicum annum: contains Apsaicine, Capsacutin, Capsaicin, Capsico
Uses. Circulatory stimulant. Induces perspiration. Infections. Intestinal disorders. Reduce clotting in blood vessels (thromboembolism). Stimulates digestion. Toothache. "Upset stomach." External. Counter- irritation applied over inflamed or irritated joint. Pain of herpes zoster ("shingles"). Condiment.
Side effects. Diarrhea, regular or bloody. Nausea. Vomiting. Vomiting blood.
Interactions. None reported.
Overdose. Diarrhea, regular or bloody. Nausea. Vomiting, vomiting blood

Caraway Carum carvi: contains Carveo Carvone, as volatile oils Calcium oxalate, Dihydro-carvone, Fatty acids, Proteins
Uses. Abdominal cramps. Appetite loss. Aromatic. Bronchitis. Colds. Cough. Digestion. Fever. Gas. Improve milk production. Induce menstruation. Liver and gallbladder problems. Memory. Nausea. Scabies. Sore throat. Tendency to infection. Used in food.
Side effects. None reported.
Interactions. None reported.
Overdose. Depression of central nervous system. Nausea. Vomiting. Kidney or liver damage

Cardamom Elettaria cardamomum, Amonum cardamonum: contains Dipentene, Fixed oil, Gum, Limonene, Terpene alcohol, Terpinene, Starch, Volatile oils, Yellow coloring

Uses. Appetite loss. Asthma. Bad breath. Bronchitis. Colds. Cough. Fever. Gas. Hemorrhoids. Improve bile flow. Laxative. Liver and gallbladder problems. Sore throat. Stomach problems. Tendency to infection.
Viruses.

Side effects. Explosive, watery diarrhea. Gallstone attack.
Interactions. None reported.
Overdose. Diarrhea. Nausea. Vomiting.

Cascara Rhamnus purshiani cortex, Cascara sagrada, sacred bark, Bitter bark, California Buckthorn, Chittem Bark, Dogwood Bark, Purshiana Bark, Yellow bark: contains Anthraquinone Cascarosides, hydroxyan thraquinone glycosides, cascarosides, resins, tannins, lipids.

Uses. Anal fissures. Hemorrhoids. Herpes simplex. Laxative. Post-anal or rectal surgery. Over-the-counter laxatives like Doxidan and Peri-colace.

Side effects. Weakened colon. Laxative dependence. Do not take with an intestinal obstruction, appendicitis, abdominal pain of unknown origin, or an inflammatory intestinal disorder. Intestinal spasms. Pain. Bloody diarrhea. Kidney irritation. Nausea. Can decrease Potassium and sodium, needed for normal heart and muscle function. Irregular heart rhythms. Bone deterioration.
Interactions. Do not take with potassium-depleting medications, like Thiazide diuretics (HydroDIURIL), steroid medications (prednisone, Deltasone), licorice root. Do not take with digoxin (Lanoxin) or a medication for heart irregularities.

Overdose. None reported. It would be reasonable to assume an exaggeration of side effects.

Castor Oil Ricinus communis, bean, Mexico castor Seed, Oil Plant, Palma Christi
Uses. Boils. Digestive ailments. Dry stool. Facial paralysis. Indigestion. Intestinal inflammation. Joint pain. Migraine. Ulcers. Worms. External. Skin inflammation. Boils. Abscesses. Earache (otitis media).
Side effects. Not to be taken with nausea, vomiting, an intestinal blockage, appendicitis, severe inflammatory intestinal disease, or any abdominal pain of unknown origin. Laxative dependence. Can deplete minerals, particularly potassium. Allergic skin rash. increase Interactions. Decreased potassium can to heart medications. Do not take with heart sensitivity medications.
Overdose. Stomach irritation. Nausea. Vomiting. Cramps. Severe diarrhea. Beans are extremely poisonous.
Severe fluid loss. Circulatory collapse.

Catalpa Catapla bignoniodes: contains Catalpin Catalposide
Uses. Antiseptic. Asthma. Bronchitis.
Gastrointestinal irritation. Parasites. Sedative.
Side effects. None reported.
Interactions. None reported.
Overdose. Sudden blood pressure drop. Faintness. Cold sweat. Paleness. Rapid pulse. Cold clammy skin. Diarrhea. Nausea. Vomiting.

Catechu Acacia catechu, black: Cutch, Catechu
contains tannins

Uses. Antiseptic. Astringent. Chronic Bleeding. diarrhea. Colitis. Decrease unusual bleeding. Diabetes. Diarrhea. Gingivitis. Mouth inflammation. Prevent secretion of fluids. Skin diseases. Sore throat.
Toothaches.

Side effects. Diarrhea. Kidney damage. Blood in urine. Decreased urine flow. Swelling of hands and feet. Vomiting.

Interactions. None reported.

Overdose. None reported. It would be reasonable to assume an exaggeration of side effects.

Khat Catha edulis: contains Cathidine, Chathine (a form of ephedrine) Celastrin, choline, Ratine

Uses. Decrease appetite. Fatigue. Stimulates brain and spinal cord.

Side effects. Increase high blood pressure. Habit forming. Addicts become talkative and then depressed and apathetic.

Interactions. None reported.

Overdose. Breathing difficulties. Depression. Euphoria. Increased blood pressure. Increased heart rate. Paralysis. Stomach irritation and bleeding.

Catnip Nepeta cataria, Catmint, Catswort, Field Balm, Monoterpene (similar to valepotriates in valerian): contains monoterpenes, acetic acid, buteric acid, citral, dipentene, lifronella, limonene, nepetalic acid, tannins, terpene, valeric acid, volatile oils.

Uses. Anemia. Boils. Bruises. Colic. Calming effects. Colds. Cramps. Coughs. Cancer. Corns. Diarrhea. Flatulence Fever Headache. Hives. Improve sleep. Indigestion. Menstrual regulation. Migraines. Muscle spasm. Nervous disorders. Parasites. Promote perspiration.

Sedative. Stimulate central nervous system. Stomachache. Teething. Toothache.

Side effect. None reported.

Interactions. None reported.

Overdose. None reported.

Catclaw Acacia, Australian Wattle

Uses. Astringent. Cough. Diaper rash. Diarrhea. Eye infection. Sore throat. Sedative. Stomachache.

Side effects. None reported.

Interactions. Anticoagulant properties. Do not take with Warfarin, Coumadin or Heparin.

Overdose. None reported.

Cat's claw Uncaria tomentosa: contains Oxyindole alkaloids

Uses. Acne. AIDS. Anti- inflammatory. Antioxidant. Arthritis. Asthma Infection. Birth control. Cancer. Depression. Diabetes. Dysentery. Gastric ulcers. Hemorrhoids. Infections. Inflammation. Inflammatory bowel disorders. Intestinal complaints. Menstrual disorders. Premenstrual syndrome. Rheumatism. Stimulate immune system. Tumors. Viral diseases. Wound healing.

Side effects. Do not take with an autoimmune illness' multiple sclerosis and tuberculosis. Do not take with organ or tissue transplants.

Interactions. Do not combine with hormonal drugs ' blood pressure medications, insulin or vaccines.

Overdose. None reported.

Cat's Foot Antennaria dioica, cudweed, Life Everlasting

Uses. Digestive problems. Ease spasms. Improve blood flow. Increase urine output.

Side effects. None reported.

Interactions. None reported.

Overdose. None reported

Cattail Typha Latifolia

Uses. Anti- inflammatory. Boils. Burn. Diarrhea. Diaper rash. Food. Kidney stones.

Side effects. Eating pollen could be dangerous for people with allergies.

Interactions. None reported.

Overdose. None reported.

Cayenne Capsicum annuum, Capsicum frutescens : contains capsaicin.

Uses. Alcoholism. Antioxidant. Atherosclerosis. Bursitis. Cramping pains. Diarrhea. Fever. Gas. Improve circulation. Indigestion. Itching. Loss of appetite. Malarial fever. Reduce platelet stickiness. Seasickness. Yellow fever. External. Counterirritant on the skin. Relieves pain. Muscular tension. Pain of diabetic neuropathy. Painful muscle spasms. Phantom pain following amputation. Rheumatism. Shingles. Stomachaches.

Side effects. Internal. Cramps. Diarrhea. Gastroenteritis. Liver damage. External. Allergic reaction. Blisters. Mild burning. Severe burning in sensitive areas. Skin inflammation. Ulcers. Keep away from the eyes and mucous membranes.

Interactions. None reported.

Overdose. Can cause a life-threatening decline in body temperature. Chronic stomach problems. Kidney damage. Liver damage. Nerve problems.

Celandine Chelidonium majus, Tetterwort
Uses. Angina. Appetite loss. Asthma. Breast lumps. Chest pain. Cramps. Gout. Hardening of the arteries. Liver and High blood pressure. Intestinal polyps. gallbladder problems. Skin conditions. Stomach cancer. Stomach problems. Water retention. Warts.
Side effects. None reported.
Interactions. None reported.
Overdose. Nausea. Vomiting. Bloody diarrhea. Blood in the urine. Stupor.

Celery Apium Graveolens: contains D-limonene, nitrates, resin, sedanoloid, sedanoic, anhydrides, volatile oils

Uses. Antioxidant. Aphrodisiac. Arthritis. Dysmenorrhea (menstrual cramps). Gas. Muscle spasm. Reduced blood pressure. Sedated.
Side effects. Skin rashes.
Interactions. Do not take with Tegretol or Tetracycline.
Overdose. Deep sedation. Premature labor.

Centaury Centaurium umbellatum, Bitter Clover, Bitterbloom, Christ's Ladder, Feverwort, Wild, Succory: contains amarogentin, erytaurin, erythrocentaurin, entiopicrin, gentisin.
Uses. Appetite loss. Diabetes. Fever. High blood pressure. Indigestion. Inflammation. Kidney stones. Malaria. Snakebite and poisoning. Stimulates saliva and digestive juices. Worms.
Side effects. Do not take if you have can't ulcer.

Interactions. None reported.
Overdose. Nausea. Vomiting.

Chamomile Anthemis Flores, A. nobilis, Matricaria appreciate you thinkingrecutita, volatile oil: contains alpha-bisabolol, oxides A & B, matricin, (converts to chamazulene), bioflavonoids, apigenin, luteolin, quercetin, antheme, anthemic acid, anthesterol, apigenin, chamazulene, resin, tannic acid, tiglic acid, volatile oils.

Uses. Anti-inflammatory. Anti-spasmodic. Appetite loss. Aromatic. Bronchitis. Burns. Colds. Cough. Cramps. Diarrhea. Fever. Gas. Indigestion. Liver and gallbladder problems. Skin inflammation. Sore throat. Tendency to infection. Wounds. External. Poultice. Skin abscesses. Kills bacteria on skin

Side effects. Irritate mucous membranes. Rare allergic reactions include bronchial constriction. Increase bleeding tendency. external. Skin reactions. In daisy family, avoid if allergic to ragweed, aster and chrysanthemum.

Interactions. Blood thinners and aspirin.

Overdose. Allergic reactions. If sensitive to ragweed pollens (rare) may have life-threatening anaphylaxis. Immediate, severe itching. Paleness. Low blood pressure. Loss of consciousness. Coma. Skin irritation. Vomiting.

Chaste Tree Vitex angus-castus
Uses. Bronchitis. Cough. Diarrhea. Low back pain. Poor circulation. Sore throat. Upper respiratory disorders. Whooping cough.

Side effects. None reported.
Interactions. None reported.
Overdose. Number ported

Chestnut Castanea sativa, Spanish Chestnut, Sweet Chestnut
Uses. Bronchitis. Cough. Diarrhea. Low back pain. Poor circulation. Sore throat. Upper respiratory disorders. Whooping cough.
Side effects. None reported
Interactions. None reported.
Overdose. None reported.

Chickweed Stellaria media, Adder's Mouth, Passerina, Satin Flower, Starweed, Stitchwort, Tongue-grass, potash salts, Rutin, flavonoids
Uses. Anti-inflammatory. Asthma. Blood disease. Constipation. Diuretic. Expectorant. Gastrointestinal disorders. Gout. Indigestion. Itching. Joint stiffness. Nose bleed. Scurvy. Skin disease. Snake bite. Sore throat. Splinters. Thin mucus in longs. Tuberculosis. Vitamin C supplements. External. Eczema. Eye. inflammation. Eyewash. Hemorrhoids. Psoriasis. Skin diseases. Wounds and burns.

Chicory Cichorium intybus, Hendibeh, Succory contains Ascorbic acid (Vitamin C), Inulin, Vitamin A
Uses. Appetite loss. Diuretic. Headache. Increasing bile flow. Indigestion. Inflammation. Kidney inflammation. Liver and gallbladder problems. Malaria. Skin allergies. Sore throat.
Side effects. Sensitivity to skin contact
Interaction. None reported
Overdose. None reported.

China Orange Citrus sinensis, Citrus dulcis, Sweet orange
Uses. Appetite loss. Calms stomach. Indigestion.
Side effects. None reported.
Interactions. None reported.

Overdose. None reported.

Chinese Cinnamon Cinnamomum aromaticum, bastard cinnamon, Cassia, False Cinnamon
Uses. Antibacterial. Appetite loss. Bedwetting. Bronchitis. Colds. Controls and growth of fungi. Cough. Diarrhea. Exhaustion. Failure to menstruate. Fever. Impotence. Improve immunity. Improved intestinal activity. Indigestion. Inhibit ulcers. Menopause. Promote weight gain. Rheumatism. Sore throat. Tendency to infection. Testicle hernia.
Side effects. Sensitivity to the herb.
Interactions. None reported
Overdose. Never reported

Chinese Foxglove Root Rehmannia Glutinosa
Uses. Blurred vision. Chronic fever. Constipation. Hearing problems. Hot flashes. Insomnia. Light-headedness. Low back pain. Menstrual irregularity. Night sweats. Palpitations. Restlessness. Stiff joints. Uterine bleeding.

Chinese Rhubarb Canton Rhubarb, Shensi Rhubarb, Rheum officinalis, R. palmatum: contains Aloe-emodin Anthraquinone Chrysophanol Emodin Tannins
Uses. Diarrhea. Prevent secretion of fluids. Shrink tissue.
Side effects. Irritate mucous membranes of intestinal tract.
Interactions. May interfere with the absorption of vitamins, minerals or medications.
Overdose. Cramping, abdominal pain. Explosive, watery diarrhea

Chondroitin contains Complex protein molecules

Uses. Anti-inflammatory. Cancer. Gout. Headaches. Improve cardiovascular health. Joint pain. Lower cholesterol levels. Lower triglyceride levels. Osteoarthritis. Prolong clotting time. Rebuild damage cartilage. Respiratory alignments. Respiratory allergies. Slow effects of aging. Wound healing. Treat torn ligaments and tendons. Most effective when combined with glucosamine sulfate

Side effects. No guarantee to the store complete mobility.

Interactions. Don't take with bleeding problems, aspirin or blood thinners, such as Coumadin.

Overdose. None reported

Cinchona Cinchona pubescens, Jesuit's Bark, Peruvian Bark

Uses. Appetite loss. Bacterial infections. Cancer. Chronic dysentery. Delay clotting. Enlarged spleen. Excessive bloating. Fever. Glue. Gas. Gout. Heartbeat irregularities. Indigestion. Irritability. Kidney inflammation. Leg ulcers. Malaria. Muscle cramps. Scrapes. Stimulates production of saliva and gastric juices

Side effects. Eczema. Itching.

Interactions. Do not take with aspirin, Coumadin or Heparin.

Overdose. Nausea. Headache. Drop in body temperature. Irregular heartbeat. Buzzing in the ears. Hearing and visual disorders including deafness and blindness. Heart failure. Asphyxiation.

Cinnamon Cinnamomum verum

Uses. Antibacterial. Antifungal. Appetite loss. Bronchitis. Cancerous tumors. Chills. Colds. Cough. Dental pain. Diarrhea. Fever. Heart problems. Hemorrhage. Improve digestion. Indigestion. Influenza. Sore throat. Tendency to infection. Urinary problems. Worm infestation. External. Cleaning wounds. Insecticide.

Side effects. Can cause a reaction. Do not confuse with other varieties

Interactions. None reported
Overdose. None reported

Cinnamon Campor, Hon-Sho, Cinnamonum camphora: contains Camphor Oil, Cineol, Cinnamaldehyde, Fatty acids, Gum, Limonene, Mannitol, Safrole, Tannins, Oils
Uses. Flavoring. Gas. Prevent secretion of fluids. Shrink tissues. A plasticizer to make celluloid explosives and other chemicals
Side effects. Nausea. Vomiting. Safrole is a possible carcinogen.
Interactions. May interfere with the absorption of vitamins, minerals or medications
Overdose. Convulsions. Dizziness. Hallucinations. Kidney damage. Coma. External. Redness. Burning sensation.

Citronella Cymbopogon species, Lemongrass
Uses. Astringent. Fragrance. Gas. Indigestion. Insect repellent. Loss of appetite. Throat problems. Worms.
Side Effects. Allergic reactions. Inhaled vapors could cause long term problems.
Interactions. None reported.
Overdose. None reported

Clivers Cleavers, Gallium aparine, Barweed, Bedstraw, Catchweed, Goose Grass, Grip Grass, Hayruff, Hedge-burs, Scratch weed, Stick-a-back
Uses. Antiseptic. Astringent. Bladder inflammation. Blood in urine. Brest lumps. Burns. Constipation. Deep-seated skin infections (carbuncles). Difficult urination. Diuretic. Edema. Gallstones. Gastritis. Infected glands. Kidney and bladder stones. Poison oak.

Skin disorders. Stomach bloating. Ulcers. Urinary tract infections. Wounds.

Side Effects. None reported.
Interactions. None reported.
Overdose. None reported.

Clover Sweet Melilotus
Uses. Antibiotic, Anti-inflammatory. Antiseptic. Aromatherapy. Arthritis. Blood thinner. Boils. Depression. Diuretic. Emollient. Expectorant. Flatulence. Headache. Sedative.
Side Effects. Vomiting
Interactions. Reduce clotting. Do not take with blood thinners like Coumadin.
Overdose. None reported. It would be reasonable to assume an exaggeration of side effects.

Cloves Syzygium Aromaticum
Uses. Antibacterial. Anti-inflammatory. Antoseptic. Aromatherapy. Arthritis. Blood thinner. Boils. Depression. Diuretic. Emollient. Expectorant. Flatulence. Headache. Sedative.
Side Effects. Irritate mucous membranes. Allergic reactions.
Interactions. None reported.
Overdose. None reported.

Cocoa Theobroma, Cacao, Chocolate
Uses. Diabetes. Diarrhea. Dilate blood vessels. Diuretic. Intestinal infections. Liver and gallbladder disorders. Muscle relaxant. Open air passages. strengthen heartbeat. Urinary tract infections.
Side effects. Migraines. Allergic reaction.
Interactions. None reported.

Overdose. Over-excitability. Racing pulse. Sleep disorders. Constipation.

Coconut Cocus nucifera: contains Fixed oil, Tannins, Trilaurin, Trimyristin, Triolein, Tripalma tic acid,
Tripalmatin, Tristearin
  Uses. Kill intestinal parasites. Prevent secretion of fluids. Relieve toothache. Shrink tissues. External. Soaps. Scalp applications. Hand creams. Foodstuffs.
  Side effects. Diarrhea
  Interactions. None reported.
  Overdose. None reported.

Coenzyme Q10
  Uses. Alzheimer's disease. Angina. Allergies. Atherosclerosis. Bell's palsy. Congestive heart failure. Diabetes. Fatigue. Huntington's disease. Improve immune System. Increase energy. Irregular heartbeat. Lower blood pressure. Meniere's disease. Muscular dystrophy.
Retinal deterioration. Weak heart.
  Side effects. None reported. Not a cure.
Interactions. None reported.
Overdose. None reported.

Coffee Charcoal, Coffea arabica
  Uses. Diarrhea. Diuretic. Increase the force of muscular contractions. Increase production of digestive juices. Mental fatigue. Migraine headache. Nerve pain. Nervousness. Physical fatigue. Relax the blood vessels (except in the brain). Relax the bronchial airways. Sore throat. Boost the effectiveness of various painkillers, including Excedrin, Vanquish, Fiorinal, Fioricet, Esgic, Wigraine, and BC Powder.

Side effects. Acid stomach. Aggravate heart condition, overactive thyroid or tendency to convulsions. Aggravate kidney disease. Anxiety or panic attacks. Diarrhea. Increase blood pressure. Increase heart rate. Physical dependence. Poor appetite. Stomach irritation. Withdrawal symptoms include headache and sleeping disorders.

Interactions. May interfere with the absorption of vitamins, minerals or medications.

Overdose. Restlessness. Irritability. Sleeplessness. Palpitations. Dizziness. Vomiting. Diarrhea. Loss of appetite. Headache. Stiffness. Muscle spasms. Rapid, irregular heartbeat. Vomiting. Abdominal spasms.

Cohosh, Black Cimicifuga racemosa, Black snake root, Bugbane, Rattle root, Richweed, Squaw root: contains tri terpene glycosides , acetin and cimicfugoside isoflavones, formononetin aromatic acids , isoferulic acid, oleic acid, palmitic acid, tannins, resins, fatty acids, starches and sugars, macrotin, xylosides acteirll and 27 -deoxyacteine

Uses. Anti-Inflammatory. Arthritis. Coughs. Decrease hot flashes. Diarrhea. Estrogen-like activity. Fever. Premenstrual discomfort. Rattlesnake bites. Sedative.

Side effects. Abdominal pain. Bradycardia. Diarrhea. Headache. Impaired digestive
Dizziness. function. Indigestion. Irritated gastrointestinal system. Joint pain. Limb pains. Low blood pressure. Nausea. Stomach discomfort. Tremors. Visual dimness. Vomiting.
cautious if taking hormone replacement or have a breast cancer history.

Interactions. Do not take with barbiturates, valium type medications or alcohol. Do not take with blood pressure medications.

Overdose. None reported. It would be reasonable to assume an exaggeration of side effects.

Cohosh, Blue Papoose Root, Squaw Root: contains Caulophyllum thalictroides, Leontin (a saponin), Methylcystine, Coulosaponin
    Uses. Menstrual problems. Raises blood pressure.
    Side effects. Chest pain. Convulsions. Dilated pupils. Headache. High blood pressure. Nausea. Stomach irritation including possible bleeding.
    Interactions. Do not take with calcium channel blockers. Do not take with nicotine patches.
    Overdose. Thirst. Vomiting. Weakness.

Cohosh, White Actaea alba, A. arguta: contains Glycosides, Protoanemonin, Volatile Oils
    Uses. Anxiety. Menstruation. Sedative.
    Side effects. Bloody diarrhea. Diarrhea. Eye irritation on contact. Hallucinations. Irritates mucous membranes. Nausea. Skin rashes. Vomiting.
    Interactions. None reported.
    Overdose. None reported. It would be reasonable to assume an exaggeration of side effects.

Cola Nut Cola acuminate, Bissy Nut, Gurru Nut, Kola Tree: contains common caffeine, theophylline
    Uses. Diuretic. Fatigue. Morning sickness. Mental Fatigue. Migraine. Physical fatigue. Suppress hunger. Suppress thirst. External. Compresses. Wounds. Inflammation.
    Side effects. Difficulty falling asleep . Excitability. Racing heart. Restlessness. Stomach

complaints. Worsen osteoporosis.

Interactions. None reported.

Overdose. None reported. It would be reasonable to assume an exaggeration of side effects.

Colchicum Colchicum autumnale, Autumn Crocus, Meadow Saffron

Uses. Decrease occurrences of gout attacks. Gout. Gout pain. Ingredient in prescription medication. Mediterranean fever.

Side effects. Bone marrow damage. Hair loss. Kidney and liver damage. Muscle diseases. Nerve inflammation.

Interactions. None reported.

Overdose. Can be extremely poisonous. Asphyxiation. Bladder spasms. Blood in the urine. Burning sensation of mouth. Circulatory collapse. Diarrhea. Difficult swallowing. Exhaustion. Fall in blood pressure. Intense thirst. Nausea. Progressive paralysis. Severe stomach pains. Vomiting.

Coltsfoot Tusilago farfara, Ass's Foot, British Tobacco, Bullsfoot, Coughwort, Donnhove, Flower Velurel Horse-Hoof, Caoutchouc: contains Pectin, Resin, Tannins, Volatile oils

Uses. Bronchitis. Coat mucous membranes to protect from irritants. Cough. Prevent secretion of fluid. Shrink tissues. Sore throat. External use: Soothe skin disorders.

Side effects. Liver damage. Has potential to cause cancer.

Interactions. None reported. May interfere with the absorption of vitamins, minerals or medications.

Overdose. None reported. It would be safe to assume an exaggeration of side effects.

Comfrey Symphytum officinale, Ass Ear, Black Root, Blackwort, Boneset, Bruisewort, Consolida, Consound, Gum Plant, Knitbone, Salsify, Slippery Root, Wallwort: contains Allantoin, Consolidine, Mucilage, Phosphorous, potassium, Pyrrolizidine, Starch, Symphyto-cynglossine, Tannins, Vitamins A and C.

Uses. Chest congestion. Diarrhea. Diuretic. Enhance tissue formation on edges of a bone fracture. Inflammation of the lungs. Laxative. Rheumatism. Stimulates reproduction of cells. Stomachache. Ulcers. Wounds and ulcers. External. Abrasions. Blunt injuries. Bruises. Dislocations. Gargle. Gum disease. Mouthwash. Prevent secretion of fluids. Reduce inflammation. Reduce swelling. Shrink tissues. Sore throat. Sprains.

Side effects. Internal. May expose to cancer-causing compounds. Coma. Drowsiness. Lethargy.

Interactions. None reported.

Overdose. None reported. Has pyrrolizidine compounds that caused cancer in animals. Liver damage. It is reasonable to assume an exaggeration of side effects.

Condurango Marsdenia condurango, Eagle Vine

Uses. Appetite loss. Enhance production of saliva and digestive juices. Indigestion. Potential for ability to kill tumors.

Side effects. None reported.

Interactions None reported.

Overdose. None reported.

Coriander Coriandrum sativum

Uses. Appetite loss. Bactericidal. Bad breath. Bladder complaints. Chest pains. Childbirth complications. Coughs. Diarrhea. Fever. Fungicidal. Gas. Headaches. Heartburn. Hemorrhoids.

Indigestion. Leprosy. Measles. Mouth and throat disorders. Rash. Rectal prolapse. Vomiting. Stimulate digestive juices Stomach and intestinal cramps.

Side effects. Sensitivity to herb.
Interactions. None reported.
Overdose. None reported.

Cornflower Centaurea cyanus, Bachelor's Buttons, Bluebonnet
Uses. Antibacterial. Colds. Eczema. Eye inflammation. Fever. Indigestion. Liver and gallbladder complaints. Menstrual disorders. Vaginal yeast infections. Water retention.
Side effects. Allergic reaction.
Interactions. None reported.
Overdose. None reported.

Corn Poppy Papaver rhoeas, Copperose, Corn Rose, Cup-Puppy, Headwark, Red Poppy
Uses. Bronchitis. Colds. Coughs. Painkiller. Sedative.
Side effects. Fresh leaves and blossoms could be poisonous. Stomach pain. Vomiting.
Interactions. None reported.
Overdose. None reported. It would be reasonable assume an exaggeration of side effects.

Cottonwood Balm of Gilead, Populus deltoides, P. candicans, P. spp silocin
Uses. Anti-inflammatory. Arthritis. Fever. Heart diseases. Pain. Toothache.
Side effects. Coma. Confusion. Convulsion.
Interactions. None reported.

Overdose. Coma. Confusion. Convulsion.

Couch Grass Agropyrum repens, Elymus repens, cutch, Dog-grass, Durfa Grass, Quack Grass, Quick Grass, Triticum, Twitch-grass, Witch grass: contains Dextrose (simple sugar), Gum, Inosite, Lactic acid, Levulose (simple sugar), Mannite, Silica, Vannilin
  Uses. Antimicrobial. Bronchitis. Chronic skin problems. Colds. Constipation. Cough. Diuretic. Fever. Gout. Improves immune system. Rheumatism. Sore throat. Urinary stones. Urinary tract infections.
  Side effects. Avoid with heart or kidney problems. Can be contaminated with ergot. Ergot cause coma, constricted blood vessels, diarrhea, itching, rapid weak pulse, spasm of the uterus, thirst, tingling, and vomiting.
  Interactions. None reported.
  Overdose. None reported. It would be reasonable to assume an exaggeration of side effects.

Cow Parsnip Hogweed, Keck, Heracleum lanatum: contains Volatile oils
  Uses. Relax muscle spasm. Sedative. Thins mucus from lungs and bronchial tubes.
  Side effects. Depress central nervous system.
  Interactions. None reported.
  Overdose. It would be reasonable to assume an exaggeration of side effects.

Cranberry Vaccinium macrocarpon, same family as bilberry
  Uses. Bactericidal to E. coli. Keep E. coli clinging to the lining of the bladder. Prevent kidney stones and bladder gravel. Remove toxins from blood.

Side effects. None reported. Do not substitute for antibiotics for acute infections.

Interactions. None reported.

Overdose. None reported.

Cranesbill Crowfoot, Geranium macula tum: contains coloring materials, Gallic acid, Gum, Pectin, Starch, Sugar, Tannins

Uses. Astringent. Decrease nosebleeds. Diarrhea. Improve blood clotting. Kills Japanese beetles. Mouthwash. Prevent secretion of fluids. Poultice. Produce puckering. Sore throat gargle.

Side effects. Blood in urine. Decreased urine flow. Diarrhea. Kidney damage. Nausea. Swelling of hands and feet. Vomiting.

Interactions. Will decrease effectiveness of Warfarin (Coumadin).

Overdose. None reported. It would be reasonable to assume an exaggeration of side effects.

Cubeb Tailed Pepper, Java Pepper, Piper cubeba: contains Cubebic acid, Cubebin: contain Fixed oil, Gum' Resin, Sesquiterpene, alcohol, cubeb camphor, Terpenes' Volatile oils

Uses. Diuretic. Gas. Thins fluid of mucus from lungs and bronchial tubes. Urinary antiseptic.

Side effects. Nausea. Vomiting.

Interactions. None reported.

Overdose. It would be reasonable to assume exaggeration of side effects.

Cumin Cumina cyminum

Uses. Anti-infective. Cramps. Diarrhea. Gas. Improve milk production. Indigestion. Inflammation. Inhibit blood clots. Worm infestations.

Side effects. None reported.

Interactions. May prolong the action of barbiturates. May interfere with blood thinners.

Overdose. None reported.

Damiana Turnera diffusa: contains terpenes, arbutin, alkaloids, chlorophyll, Damianian, Resin, Starch, Sugar, Tannins, Volatile oils

Uses. Antidepressant. Aphrodisiac. Asthma. Bronchitis. Decreases or cures bedwetting. Euphoria-inducing. Headache. Neurosis. Sexual disorders. Purging agent.

Side effects. Euphoria. Laxative effect. Bitter taste.

Interactions. None reported.

Overdose. None reported. It would be reasonable to assume an exaggeration of side effects.

Dandelion Taraxacum officinale, Blowball, Cankerwort, Lion's Tooth, Priest 'g Crown, Swine's Snout, Wild Endive: contains bitters, fats, gluten, gum, inulin, iron, niacin, potash, potassium, proteins, resin, teraxacerin, vitamins A, C and D, sesquiterpene, lactones of eudesmanolide and germacranolide, magnesium, zinc, managanese. Related to chicory.

Uses. Anemia. Appetite loss. Blood purifiers. Diuretic Cancer. Chronic ulcers. Constipation. Diabetes. Dyspepsia. Eczema. Gout. Heart trouble. Hemorrhoids. Indigestion. Hepatitis. milk production. Inflamed breast tissue. Joint problems. Kidney and bladder stones. Liver and gallbladder problems. Poor digestion. Rheumatism. Stimulates stomach secretions • Toothache. Tuberculosis. Urinary tract infections. Warts

Side effects. Take care if you have gallstones or if bi le ducts are obstructed. Gastritis. Heartburn. Increase stomach acid. Rash. Stomach ulcers.

Interactions. Do not take with Lithium. Do not take with blood pressure medications Do not take with diuretics.

Overdose. None reported. It would be reasonable to assume an exaggeration of side effects.

Delphinium Flower Delphinium consolida, Branching Larkspur, Knight 's Spur, Lark Heel, Staggerweed

Uses. Appetite loss. Diuretic. Urinary tract infections. Worms.

Side effects. Do not overuse.

Interactions. None reported.

Overdose. None reported.

Devils Claw Harpogophytum procumbens, Grapple Plant, Wood Spider: contains members of the iridoid glycoside family, harpagoside, harpagide and procumbide

Uses. Anti- inflammatory. Appetite loss. Arthritis. High blood pressure. Increase bile production.
Indigestion. Liver and gallbladder problems. Pain. Pregnancy difficulties. Produce digestive juices.
Rheumatism. Skin disorders.

Side effects. Allergic reaction. Increase stomach acid.

Interactions. Do not take with heart medicatiOnS• with thyroid medications. Do not take with not take diuretics. Do not take with antacids.

Overdose. None reported. It would be reasonable to assume an exaggeration of side effects.

Dill Anethum graveolens

Uses. Appetite loss. Bad breath. Bronchitis. Colds. Cough. Fever. Gas. Inhibit bacteria. Kidney and urinary tract conditions. Liver and gallbladder problems. Skin diseases. Sleep disorders. Sore throat. Spasms. Stomach and intestinal problems. Tendency to infection. Upset stomach.

Side effects. Topical application can react with sunlight.

Interactions. None reported.

Overdose. None reported.

Dock Rumes: contains oxalic acid

Uses. Acne. Anemia. Antiseptic. Astringent. Bites. Boils. Burns. Cancer. Constipation. Diarrhea. Hepatitis. Menstrual problems. Parasites. Rheumatism. Sore throat.
Stinging nettle. Tumors. Venereal diseases. Wounds.

Side effects. None reported.

Interactions. Oxalic acid interferes with calcium absorption.

Overdose. None reported.

Dong Quai Dang-gui, Angelica sinensis, Female ginseng, member of the celery family

Uses. Abnormal menstruation. Antispasmodic. Arthritis. Cancer. Cardiovascular disease. Fatigue. High blood pressure. Hot flashes. Improve immune Peripheral system. Painful menstruation. Circulation. Production of red blood cells. Suppressed menstrual flow. Uterine bleeding.

Side effects. Sensitivity to sun. No estrogen or hormone-like effects.

Interactions. Do not take with blood thinners or aspirin. Do not take with estrogen. Caffeine.

Overdose. None reported

Echinacea Echinacea Purpurea, Echinacea angustifolia, purple coneflower, rudbeckia, Sampson Root

Uses. Abscesses. Bites. Bronchitis. Burns. Colds. Cough. Earache. Fever.
Improve immune system. Improve Flu. Gonorrhea. Herpes. Infection. white blood cells after cancer treatments. Measles. Mouth ulcers. Septicemia. Skin problems. Snake bite. Sore throat. Speed wound healing. Stomach cramps. Swelling of the lymph nodes. Tendency to infection. Tuberculosis. Tumors. Urinary tract infections. Viruses.

Side effects. Do not take if you have autoimmune illness, cancer, AIDS, HIV, or on immunosuppressant therapy, tuberculosis or multiple sclerosis. Be careful if allergic to the daisy family. Fever. Gastrointestinal distress. Headache. Nausea. Vomiting. Don't take injections if you have diabetes. Injections may cause shivers, short-term fever, or an immediate allergic reaction.

Interactions. Liver damage in combination anabolic steroids or methotrexate. Decrease effect of corticosteroids.

Overdose. None reported. It would be reasonable to assume an exaggeration of side effects.

Elderberry Sambucus nigra, Sambucus canadensis, Black Elder, Boor Tree, Bountry, Ellanwood, Ellhorn, European Alder: contains albumin, cyanide, flavonoids, quercetin, itydrocyanic acid, resin, rutin, sambucine, sambunigrin, tannic acid, tyrosin, viburnic acid, Viatmin C, volatile oils, wax

Uses. Abdominal pain. Anti-inflammatory. Arthritis. Bronchitis. Bruises. Colds. Cough. Diuretic. Fevers. Headache. Increase perspiration. Gout. Infections. Inhibit viruses. Laxative. Menstrual cramps.
Pain relief. Poultice. Purging effect. Sore throat. Sprain. Upper respiratory ailments.

Side effects. Irritate gastrointestinal tract. Vomiting.
Interactions. None reported.
Overdose. Abdominal pain. Diarrhea. Nausea. Stems have cyanide and are toxic. Vomiting.

Elecampane Inula Helenium, Elfdock, Horse-Elder, Horseheal, Scabwort, Velvet Dock, Wild Sunflower
Uses. Bactericidal. Bronchitis. Cough. Diarrhea. Fungicidal. Gas. Gallbladder problems. Inflammation. Intestinal inflammation. Menstrual complaints. Loosen phlegm in the lungs. Upset stomach. Vomiting. Water retention.
Side effects. Irritate the lining of the nose, throat, stomach, and intestines. Allergic reaction.
Interactions. None reported.
Overdose. Diarrhea. Paralysis. Spasms. Vomiting.

Eleuthero Eleutherococcus senticosus, Acanthopanax senticosus, Siberian ginseng, ci wu ju, touch-me-not, devils shrub, related to Asian ginseng: contains eleutherosides B and E and complex polysaccharides
Uses. Autoimmune illnesses. Chronic fatigue syndrome. Colds. Combat harmful toxins. Decrease infections. function. Endurance. Immune Energy. HIV. Improve Respiratory tract infections. Stamina. Stress-related illness. Vitality.
Side effects. Mild diarrhea. Insomnia. Do not take if You have uncontrolled high blood pressure.
Interactions. Do not take with blood thinners or aspirin. Do not take with diabetic medications.
Overdose. None reported. It would be reasonable to assume an exaggeration of side effects.

English Ivy Hedera helix, Common Ivy, Gum Ivy, True Ivy, Woodbind

Uses. Bronchitis. Cough. Expectorant. Gout. Inflamed lymph nodes. Liver, spleen and gallbladder disorders. Rheumatism. External. Burns. Calluses. Inflamed veins. Inflammation. Nerve pain. Parasites. Ulcers.

Side effects. Allergic skin reactions to leaves.

Interactions. None reported.

Overdose. None reported.

English Oak Quercus robur, Tanner's Bark

Uses. Anti-inflammatory. Astringent. Bronchitis. Colds. Cough. Diarrhea. Fever. Skin inflammation. Sore throat. Tendency to infection.

Side effects. Internal. Digestive problems. External. Do not use on open skin lesions. Do not use if you have fever, infection or a weak heart.

Interactions. Interferes with absorption of morphine, quinine, nicotine, and caffeine.

Overdose. None reported. It would be reasonable to assume an exaggeration of side effects.

English Plantain Plantago Lanceolata, Buckhorn, Chimney-sweeps, Headsman, Ribwort, Ripplegrass, Soldier's Herb

Uses. Antibacterial. Astringent action. Bronchitis. Burns. Colds. Cough. Fever. Sore Skin inflammation. throat. Stop bleeding. Tendency to infection • Upper respiratory tract infection. Wounds.

Side effects. None reported.

Interactions. Do not take with blood thinners or aspirin. May interfere with absorption of medications.
Do not take with Lithium or Tegretol (carbamazepine).

Overdose. None reported.

Ephedra Ephedra, Ephedra sinica, Ephedra Intermedia, Ephedra equisetina, Ma huang, Chinese Joint Fir: contains ephedrine and pseudophedrine.

Uses. Asthma. Bactericidal. Bone pain. Bronchial spasms. Bronchitis. Common cold. Congestion. Cough. Elevate blood pressure. Fevers without sweat. Increase heart rate. Lung and bronchial constriction. Obesity. Relieve sweating. Stimulate the CNS. Water retention. Weight loss. Main component in Primatene Tablets.

Side effects. Anxiety. Dry mouth. Disrupt heart rhythm. Headache. Heart failure. Heart palpitations. High blood pressure. Insomnia. Irritability. Muscle disturbances. Nausea. Nervousness. Rapid heartbeat.
Restlessness. Sleeplessness. Urinary disorders. Vomiting. Do not take with diabetes, glaucoma, heart conditions, high blood pressure, overactive adrenal gland, prostate cancer, thyroid disease, or weakened blood vessels in the brain. Do not drive or operate machinery if taking pseudoephedrine.

Interactions. Disturbance of heart rhythm with digoxin (Lanoxin). Increase stimulating effects taken with the blood pressure medication guanethidine Do not (Ismelin), or Eldepryl (Parkinson's medication). i.e. Nardil take with MAO inhibiting antidepressants, and Parnate. Can cause high blood pressure if taken with migraine medications i.e. Ergomar and Wigraine, or with heart medications Okytocin. Do not take if on, decongestants, or theophylline. Enlarged pupils. Spasms.

Overdose. Severe sweating. Life- threatening. Heart Increased body temperature.
failure. Suffocation.

Eryngo Eryngium campestre, Sea Holly, Sea Holme, Sea Hulver
Uses. Bronchitis. Colds. Coughs. Difficulty urinating. Diuretic. Gas. Kidney and urinary tract inflammation. Kidney pain. Loosen phlegm. Prostate. Skin disorders. Spasms. Urinary tract infections. Water retention.
Side effects. None reported.
Interactions. None reported.
Overdose. None reported.

Eucalyptus Eucalyptus globulus, Blue Gum, Red Gum
Uses. Acne. Asthma. Bactericide. Bad breath. Bladder, liver, and gallbladder conditions. Bleeding gums. Bronchitis. Cough. Diabetes. Decongestant. Digestive complaints. Fever. Flu. Fungicide. Gonorrhea. Headache. Hoarseness. Loosens phlegm. Loss of appetite. Measles. Nerve pain. Poorly healing sores. Rheumatism. Scarlet fever. Sinus conditions. Sore mouth. Spasms. Threadworm. Tuberculosis. Whooping cough. Worms. Wounds. External. Improves local circulation. Ingredient in Listerine antiseptic Mouth rinse, Mentholatum Cherry Chest Rub, and Vicks VaporRub.
Side effects. Do not take with digestive problems. Bile duct or liver disease. Asthma-like symptoms. Nausea. Vomiting. Diarrhea.
Interactions. None reported.
Overdose. Poisoning. Drop in blood pressure. Circulation problems. Collapse. Asphyxiation.

European Buckthorn Rhamnus frangula, Arrow Wood, Black Alder, Frangula Bark, Persian Berries
Uses. Surgery. Constipation. Hemorrhoids. Soften stool. Stimulates contractions of the intestinal wall.

Side effects. Do not take with intestinal obstruction or appendicitis. Can aggravate acute inflammatory disorders of the intestines like ulcerative colitis or crohn's disease. Bone deterioration. Cramps. Decrease potassium. Kidney disease. Heart problems. Intestinal dysfunction. Swelling. Vomiting.

Interactions. Increase effects of heart medications.

Overdose. Bone deterioration. Cramps. Heart problems. Kidney disease. Swelling. Vomiting.

Evening Primrose Oil Oenothera biennis, Fever Plant, King's Cureall, Night Willow-herb, Scabish, Scurvish, Sun Drop

Uses. Alcoholism. Antiseptic. Arthritis. Asthma. Astringent. Cardiovascular diseases. Cough. Diabetes. Diarrhea. Diuretic. Eczema. High blood pressure. Hyperactivity. Inflammation. Menstrual irregularities. Migraine. Premenstrual syndrome (PMS). Reduce Ch01ester01. Sedative. Skin inflammation. Weight loss. Whooping cough. Wounds.

Side effects. None reported.

Interactions. None reported. People with schizophrenia who are taking phenothiazines are at risk for interactions, may cause seizures.

Overdose. Headache. Nausea. Stomach pain. Temporal lobe epilepsy tendency.

Eyebright Euphrasia Officinals: contains iridoid glycosides, flavonoids, tannnins bitters, volatile oils

Uses. Astringent. Blepharitis (inflammation of the eyelids). Conjunctivitis. Coughs. Discomfort of eyestrain or minor irritation. Functional eye disorders. Hoarseness. Inflamed prostate. Irritated

eyes. Poultice for inflammations, fatigue and vis ion disturbance. Sinus infections. Sore throat. Tired eyes.
Treatment of styes.

Side effects. Do not use in eyes because is not sterile.

Interactions. None reported.

Overdose. None reported.

Fennel Foeniculm vulgare: contains Terpenoid anethole, volatile oil

Uses. Anemia. Antimicrobial. Bloating. Bronchitis. Colic. Cough. Diarrhea. Digestive problems. Diuretic. Dry respiratory phlegm. Estrogen- like activity. Fever. Gas. Heartburn. Hernia. Increase bile production.
Increase breast milk. Indigestion. Intense thirst. Intestinal spasms. Irritable bowel syndrome. Pain. Skin diseases. Stomach spasms. Upper respiratory inflammation. Vomiting.

Side effects. Do not take if have an estrogen dependent cancer. May have a cross allergy to celery.

Interactions. None reported.

Overdose. Congestive Heart failure. Nausea Vomiting.

Fenugreek Trigonella foenum-graecum, Bird's Foot: contains steroidal saponins, choline, fixed oil, iron/
lecithin, mucilage, phosphates, protein, trigonelline' trimethylamine, volatile oils

Uses. Abscesses. Appetite. Digestive Atherosclerosis. Beriberi. Constipation. High problems. Fever. Hernia. High cholesterol. triglycerides. Impotence. Increase milk production. Indigestion. Kidney problems. Male reproductive tract difficulty. Promote healing. Reduce blood sugar. Skin inflammation. Steroids. Upper respiratory inflammation. Wounds. External. Boils. Eczema. Hives. Vomiting.

Ulcers.

Side effects. Skin allergy. Take with care if diabetic.

Interactions. May interfere with absorption of medications. Do not take with diabetic drugs. Do not take with blood thinners or aspirin.

Overdose. Intestinal upset. Nausea.

Feverfew Featherfoil , Midsummer Daisy, Bachelor's Buttons, Altamisa, Chrysanthemum parthenium, tanacetum parthenium : contains sesquiterpene lactones, parthenolide, Pyrethrins, Santamarin

Uses. Allergies. Appetite loss. Arthritis. "Blood purifier." Common cold. Cramps. Decrease edema. Diarrhea. Fever. Gargle. Gas. General tonic. Improve blood vessel tone. Indigestion. Inflammation. Intestinal parasites (worms). Menstrual disorders. Migraine. Painful menstruation. Postnatal bleeding. Prevent excessive clumping of platelets. Prevent infection. Reduce swelling from wounds. Stimulate uterine contractions. Thin mucus from lungs and bronchial tubes. Tranquilizer. External. Insecticide.

Side effects. Abdominal pain. Diarrhea. Flatulence. Gastrointestinal upset. Indigestion. Loss of taste. Mouth ulcerations. Nausea. Nervousness. Rebound headache if stopped suddenly. Skin reactions. Swelling of lips, tongue and mouth. Vomiting.

Interactions. Can interfere with platelet activity and increase bleeding. Do not take with blood thinners or aspirin. Prolong clotting times.

Overdose. Do not take if allergic to pyrethrin's. Immediate, severe itching, paleness, low blood pressure, loss of consciousness, coma.

Fig Ficus carica

Uses. Constipation. Infectious diarrhea. Intestinal inflammation. Laxative effect.

Side effect. None reported.

Interactions. None reported.

Overdose. None reported.

Flaxseed Linseed, Linum usitatissimum: contains gum, fixed oil, linamarin, mucilage, protein, tannins, wax

Uses. Abrasions. Antiseptic. Boils. Burns. Constipation. Coughs. Eye infection. Gout. High cholesterol. Poultice. Rheumatism. Skin infections. Sore throat. Stomachache.

Side effects. One part of flaxseed may convert to cyanide. Convulsions. Rapid breathing. Paralysis. Unusual excitement. Weakness.

Interactions. May interfere with the absorption of medications. May cause increased flush with Niacin.

Overdose. None reported. It would be reasonable to assume an exaggeration of side effects

Fo-ti Polygonum multiflorium, He-shou-wu, white foti, if boiled red Fo-Ti

Uses. Abscesses. Angina pectoris. Antibacterial. Atherosclerosis. Blurred vision. Constipation. Deep skin infections. Dizziness. Fatigue. Goiter and neck lumps. Hardening of the arteries. High cholesterol. Immune function. Impotence. Infectious diseases. Insomnia. Nocturnal emission. Premature aging. Red blood cell formation. Sores. Sore knees and back. Weakness. Vaginal discharges.

Side effects. Unprocessed. Digestive distress. Flushing of the face. Mild diarrhea. Numb arms or legs. Skin rash.

Interactions. None reported. Do not take with onions, chives, or garlic.

Overdose. Diarrhea. Numbness in the arms or legs.

Fritillia Pei -Mu, Fritillia vericillia, F. meleagris, Frimitime: contains Fritilline, Peimine, Peiminine, verticine, Verticilline, Peimine, peiminine: resemble steroid hormones.

Uses. Decrease blood pressure. Fever. Increase breast milk. Increase blood sugar. Thin mucus of lungs and bronchial tubes.

Side effects. Adversely affect the electrical system of the heart. Heart block with rate below 50. Heartbeat irregularity.

Interactions. None reported.

Overdose. None reported. It would be reasonable to assume an exaggeration of side effects.

Frostwort Helianthemum canadense, Rock-Rose, Sun Rose Uses. Astringent. Indigestion. Skin conditions. Skin inflammation.

Uses. Astringent. Indigestion. Skin conditions. Skin inflammation.

Side effects. None reported.

Interactions. None reported.

Overdose. None reported.

Fumitory Fumaria officinalis, Beggary, Earth Smoke, Vapor

Uses. Arthritis. Bladder Infections. Liver and Clogged arteries. Gallbladder problems. Low blood sugar. skin diseases.

Side effects. None reported.

Interactions. None reported.

Overdose. None reported.

Galangal Alpinia galanga, Alpinia officinarum,

Galanga Major & Minor, Catarrh Root, China Root, Chinese Ginger, Colic Root , India Root : contains cineloe, galangin, galangol, kaempferid, resin, volatile oils

Uses. Anti-bacterial. Appetite loss. Arthritis. Bronchitis. Chronic heart disorders. Colds. Cough.
Decrease phlegm from allergies. Diabetes. Diarrhea. Difficulty swallowing. Dizziness. Fatigue. Fever. Gas. Heart pain. Impotence. Improve immune system. Indigestion. Liver and gallbladder problems. Painful teeth and gums. Sore throat. Stimulates respiration.

Side effects. Diarrhea. Nausea. Vomiting.

Interactions. None reported.

Overdose. None reported. It would be reasonable to assume an exaggeration of side effects.

Galega European Goat Rue, officinalis: contains bitters, galegine, tannins

Uses. Diabetes. Increase breast milk.

Side effects. Headache. Jitteriness. Weakness.
Interactions. None reported.

Overdose. None reported. It would be reasonable to assume an exaggeration of side effects.

Gambier Pale Catechu, Gambir, Uncaria gambier: contains catechin, catechutannic acid, tannins

Uses. Chronic diarrhea. Decrease unusual bleeding. Shrink tissues. Sore throat gargle.

Side effects. Blood in urine. Decreased urine flow. Diarrhea. Kidney damage. Swelling of hands and feet. Vomiting.

Interactions. May interfere with the absorption of vitamins, minerals and medications.

Overdose. None reported. It would be reasonable to assume an exaggeration of side effects.

Gamboge Garcinia hanburyi, Gummigutta, Gutta Gamba, Tom Rong

Uses. Constipation. Diarrhea. Hemorrhoids. Indigestion. Inflammations. Ulcers.

Side effects. Abdominal pain. Ineffective straining. Vomiting.

Interactions. None reported.

Overdose. Abdominal pain. Vomiting. Death.

Garlic Allium sativum: contains allicin, ajoene, allyl sulfides, vinyldithiins, phytoncides, unsaturated aldehydes, volatile oils

Uses. Abdominal pain. Antibacterial. Anti-cancer agent. Anti-clotting. Antifungal. Antioxidant.
Antiviral. Bronchitis. Colds. Congestive heart failure. Cough. Diabetes. Digestion. Diuretic. Fever. Hardening of the arteries. Hypercholesterolemia. Hyperlipemia. Hypertension. Improve immune function. Increase blood flow to skin. Intermittent claudication. Kill larvae. Menstrual pain. Stimulate perspiration. Sore throat. Thins from lungs and bronchial tubes. External use. Calluses. Corns. Ear infections. Muscle and nerve pain. Sciatica.

Side effects Bad breath. Body odor. Eczema. Flatulence. Heartburn. Stomach problems. Increase
bleeding time. Increase risk of bleeding during and after surgery.

Interactions. Do not take with blood thinners or aspirin. Do not take with diabetic medications.

Overdose. Increase the number of white blood cells. Skin eruptions. Blood-pressure drop. Faintness. Cold sweat. Paleness. Rapid pulse.

Gay-Feather Liatris, vanilla plant
Uses. Backache. Cough. Diuretic. Gonorrhea. Headache. Menstrual regulation. Nosebleed. Snakebite. Tonsillitis. Talisman.
Side effects. Prevent blood clotting.
Interactions. Enhance blood thinners.
Overdose. None reported. It would be reasonable to assume an exaggeration of side effects.

Gentian Gentiana lutea, Bitter Root, Bitterwort, Yellow Gentian: contains glycosides, gentiopicrin, amarogentin, gentiamarin, gentiin, gentiopicrin, gentisin, mesogentioigenin, protogentiogenin, sugar, xanthrone pigment
Uses. Antidote to certain poisons. Appetite loss. Diarrhea. Digestion. Fevers. Increase saliva. Increase stomach acid. Indigestion. Malaria. Protect the liver.
External use. Skin tumors.
Side effects. Excessive stomach acid. Gastritis. Heartburn. Nausea. Stomach ulcers. Vomiting.
Interactions. None reported.
Overdose. None reported. It would be reasonable to assume an exaggeration of side effects.

Gentiana Gentiana scabra: contains amarogentin
Uses. Antibiotic. Appetite loss. Hepatitis. Increase digestive juices. Increase saliva. Indigestion. Liver disorders. Malaria. Pain and swelling of the genital area. Pelvic inflammation. Seizures. Sexually transmitted diseases. Vaginal discharge.
Side effects. Acid. Diarrhea. Heartburn. Indigestion. Ulcer
Interactions. None reported.
overdose. None reported. It would be reasonable to assume an exaggeration of side effects.

German Chamomile Mazanilla, Matricaria, Hungarian Chamomile, Matricaria chamomilla : contains alphabisabolol, azulene, fatty acid, furfural , paraffin hydrocarbons , sesquiterpene, sesquiterpene alcohol, tannins

Uses. Anti-inflammatory. Gas. Muscle spasms. Sedative. Tonic.

Side effects. Weakens muscles. May increase bleeding.

Interactions. Do not take with blood thinners or aspirin. May interfere with the absorption of vitamins, minerals and medications. Do not take with barbiturates, valium-type medications or alcohol.

Overdose. Diarrhea. Excess sedation. Nausea. Skin eruptions. Vomiting.

German Sarsaparilla Carex arenaria, Red Couchgrass, Red Sedge, Sand Sedge, Sea Sedge

Uses. Colds. Cramps. Diabetes. Fevers. Gas. Gout. Kill insects. Liver disorders. Menstrual irregularity. Rheumatism. Skin conditions. Tuberculosis. Urinary tract infections. Venereal disease. Water retention.

Side effects. None reported. May interfere with absorption of medications.

Interactions. None reported.

Overdose. None reported.

Ginger ingiber officinale: contains 1-4% volatile oils, zingiberene, bisabolene, gingerols, shogaols, borneal, cineole, citral, sequiterpene, volatile oils, zingerone

Uses. Abdominal bloating. Appetite loss. Asthma. Atherosclerosis. Boost heart' s pumping action.

Chemotherapy support. Cough. Decrease blood platelets clumping and stickiness. Diarrhea. Earache. Gag. Loosen phlegm. Migraines. Morning sickness. Motion sickness. Nausea. Post-operative nausea and vomiting. Protect stomach from damaging effect of alcohol and medicines. Rheumatism. Rheumatoid arthritis. Sexual disorders. Shortness of breath. Tighten tissues. Ulcers. Vomiting. Water retention.

Side effects. Heartburn. May create problems with gallstones.

Interactions. Increase bleeding time. May interfere with blood thinners. May interfere with heart or diabetic medications.

Overdose. None reported.

Ginkgo Biloba Ginko biloba, maidenhair tree: contains Ginkgo flavone glycosides, terpene lactones, Ginkgolides, bilobalide

Uses. Alzheimer's disease. Antioxidant. Anxiety. Atherosclerosis. Cerebrovascular insufficiency. CHF. Circulatory disorders. Depression. Diabetes. Dizziness. Headache. Impotence/infertility (male). Improve concentration. Inhibit clots. Inhibit platelet clumping. Intermittent claudication. Macular degeneration. Migraine. Multiple sclerosis. Protect nerves. Raynaud's. Reinforce small blood vessels. Respiratory tract conditions. Ringing in the ears. Senility. Short-term memory loss.

Side effects. Allergic reaction. Cramps. Digestive problems. Headaches. Spasms. Upset stomach.

Interactions. May increase the action of blood thinners or anti-clot medicines.

Overdose. Increase bleeding time. Severe weakness Spontaneous hemorrhage.

Ginseng Panex ginseng, Arabinose, Camphor: contains Gineosides Mucilage, Panaxosides, Resin, Saponin, Starch, contains: "adaptogen"

Uses. Depression. Diabetes. Edema. Fatigue. Hardening of the arteries. Heart problems. Impotence. Improve concentration. Improve immune system. Improve mental and physical efficiency. Increase corticosteroid. Increase Indigestion. Stimulate brain, heart, blood
histamine. vessels. Stress. Ulcers. Urinary disturbances.

Side effects. Do not take with cardiovascular disease, diabetes, or high blood pressure.

Interactions. If taken with non-steroidal anti-inflammatory drugs (NSAIDS) may cause blistering and sloughing of skin (Stevens-Johnson syndrome). Increase the effects of MAO inhibitors, i.e. phenelzine (Nardil). Do not take with antidiabetic medicines, antipsychotics, blood thinners, blood pressure medications or steroids. Worsens agitation of caffeine.

Overdose. Breast pain. Diarrhea. Insomnia. Mania if taking phenelzine. Nausea. Nervousness. Post-menopausal bleeding. Sleeplessness. Tight muscles. Vomiting. Water retention.

Glucosamine

Uses. Aids formation of ligaments, and nails. Ankylosing spondylitis. Bursitis. Inflammation. Injury to the joints. Joint pain. Osteoarthritis. Promote cartilage. Rheumatoid arthritis. Spinal disc degeneration. Tendonitis. Indigestion.

Side effects. Diarrhea. Heartburn. Nausea.

Interactions. None reported.

Overdose. None reported. It would be reasonable to assume an exaggeration of side effects.

Goat's Rue Galega officinal is, French Lilac, Italian Fitch
Uses. Diuretic. Lower blood sugar.
Side effects. None reported.
Interactions. None reported.
Overdose. Spasms, paralysis, asphyxiation, death (in animals).

Goldenrod Solidago Species
Uses. Anti- inflammatory. Antiseptic. Antispasmodic. Asthma. Burns. Chest pain. Colic. Constipation. Cough. Cramps. Diabetes. Diarrhea. Diuretic. Enlarged liver. Enlarged prostate. Fever. Gas. Gout. Headache. Hemorrhoids. Internal bleeding. Kidney and bladder stones. Kidney pain. Mouth and throat infections. Measles. Respiratory conditions. Rheumatism. Snakebite. Sore throat. Toothache. Tuberculosis. Urinary tract infections. Wounds.
Side effects. Avoid with chronic kidney disease, heart or kidney problems. Do not take if allergic.
Interactions. None reported.
Overdose. None reported.

Goldenseal Hydrastis canadensis, Eye Balm, Ground Raspberry, Indian Paint, Jaundice Root, Yellow Root: contains albumin, berberine, candine, fats, hydrastine/ lignin, resin, starch, sugar, volatile oils, two primary alkaloids
Uses. Antibiotic. Anti- inflammatory. Antimicrobial. Canker sores. Crohn's disease. Decrease uterine bleeding. Depress muscle tone of small blood vessels. Dyspepsia. Improve appetite. Indigestion. Infectious diarrhea. Premenstrual syndrome (PMS) . Recurrent ear infection. Reduce blood pressure. Sore throat. Stimulate central nervous system. Upper respiratory infections. Vaginal infections. Combined with echinacea for colds and flu. External. Eye infection. Skin inflammation. Wounds.

Side effects. Breathing difficulties. Constipation. Delifium. Diarrhea. Digestive problems. Gastrointestinal distress. Hallucinations. Hypertension. Mouth and throat irritation. Nausea. Nervous excitement. Nervous system. Numbness of hands and feet. Paralysis. effects
Ulcerations. Vomiting. Weakness.

Interactions. Decrease absorption and use of vitamin B. Do not take with blood thinners or aspirin. Do not take with blood pressure medicines. Is on the protected species list.

Overdose. Difficult breathing. Edema. Hypertension. paralysis. Reduce sodium excretion. Slow heart rate. Spasms. Vomiting. Weaken good bacteria of the digestive tract.

Gotu Cola Kola, Gbanja Kola, Cola nitida: contains caffeine, catechol, epicatechol, theobromine

Uses. Astringent. Congestive heart failure. Decrease fatigue. Diuretic. High blood pressure. Increase sex drive. Prevent secretion of fluids. Stimulate central nervous system.

Side effects. Can worsen ulcers in esophagus, stomach or duodenum. Nervousness. Sleeplessness.

Interactions. Caffeine. Theophylline (Aminophylline).

Overdose. None reported. It would be reasonable to assume an exaggeration of side effects.

Gotu Kola Centella asiatica, Indian pennywort, Marsh Penny, White Rot: contains saponins (also called triterpenoids), known as asiaticoside, madecassoside and madasiatic acid

Uses. Asthma. Bronchitis. Chronic venous insufficiency. Coughs. Dehydration. Depression. Diarrhea. Dysentery. Epilepsy. Exhaustion. Eye conditions. Fever. Heart problems. High blood pressure. Hoarseness. Hysteria. Improves healing of injuries. Improve thought processes. Inflammation. Insomnia. Jaundice. Kills certain bacteria. Leg pain, heaviness, and swelling. Leprosy. Mental illness. Muscle and joint problems. Nervous disorders. Prolong life. Rheumatism. Scleroderma. Sedative. Skin ulcers. Syphilis. Ulcers. Urinary difficulties. Varicose veins. Water retention.

Side effects. Allergy. Nausea. Sedation. Skin rash.

Interactions. Do not take with barbiturates, valium type medications or alcohol.

Overdose None reported.

Grape Hyacinth Muscari racemonsum, M. comosum: contains cosmisic acid, saponin

Uses. Asthma. Bronchitis. Chronic venous insufficiency. Coughs. Dehydration. Depression. Diarrhea. Dysentery. Epilepsy. Exhaustion. Eye conditions. Fever. Heart problems. High blood pressure. Hoarseness. Hysteria. Improves healing of injuries. Improve thought processes. Inflammation. Insomnia. Jaundice. Kills certain bacteria. Leg pain, heaviness, and swelling. Leprosy. Mental illness. Muscle and joint problems. Nervous disorders. Prolong life. Rheumatism. Scleroderma. Sedative. Skin ulcers. Syphilis. Ulcers. Urinary difficulties. Varicose veins. Water retention.

Side effects. Allergy. Nausea. Sedation. Skin rash.

Interactions. Do not take with barbiturates, valium type medications or alcohol.

Overdose None reported.

Greater Burnet Sanguisorba officinalis, Garden Burnet

Uses. Coughing up of blood. Diarrhea. Difficulty urinating. Heavy menstrual flow. Hemorrhoids. Hot flashes. Infectious diarrhea. Inflammation of leg veins. Intestinal inflammation. Menopausal disorders. Nosebleed. Varicose veins.

External. Boils. Stops bleeding. Wounds.
Side effects. None reported.
Interactions. None reported.
Overdose. None reported.

Green Tea Camellia sinensis, Chinese Tea, derived from
Camellia sinensis (green, black and oolong tea):
contains volatile oils, vitamins, minerals and caffeine, tannins,
polyphenols, particularly the catechin called epigallocatechin gal late
(EGCG).
Uses. Antibacterial. Body aches and pains. Cancer. Dental
plaque. Depression. Detoxification. Diarrhea. Dizziness. Drowsiness.
Energizer. Excessive thirst. Good health. Headache. Heart pain.
Gingivitis.
Hemorrhoids. High cholesterol High triglycerides. Hypertension.
Immune function. Indigestion. Infection. Insomnia. Motion sickness.
Periodontal disease. Prolong life. Reduce platelet clumping. Stimulate
the central nervous system.
Side effects. Acid stomach. Anxiety. Constipation.
Diarrhea. Insomnia. Panic attacks. Poor appetite. Stomach irritation.
Take with care with weak heart, kidney disease, overactive thyroid or
spasms.
Interactions. Interferes with absorption of alkaline
medications. May increase the risk of miscarriage. Do not take with
calcium.
Overdose. Abdominal spasms. Diarrhea. Dizziness.
Exaggerated reflexes. Headache. Irregular heartbeat. Irritability. Loss
of appetite. Restlessness. Sleeplessness. Tremors. Vomiting.
Grindelia Gumweed, Rosinweed, Grindelia camporum, G.
humilus, G. squarrosa: contains balsamic resin, grindelol, robustic
acid, saponins, tannins, volatile, robust oils

Uses. Asthma. Bronchitis. Decrease heart rate. Dilate Pupils of eyes. Increase blood pressure. Sedative. Thin mucus from lungs and bronchial tubes. External. Burns. Poultice to apply medications. Vaginitis.

Side effects. None reported.

Interactions. May interfere with the absorption vitamins, minerals and medications.

Overdose. Blood in urine. Decreased urine flow Depress central nervous system. Kidney damage. swelling of hands and feet.

Guaiac Guaiacum officinale, Lignum Vitae, Pockwood: contains guaiaconic acid, guaiaretic acid saponin, vanillin

Uses. Arthritis. Constipation. Edema. Increase perspiration. Respiratory complaints. Rheumatism. Scrofula. Skin disorders. Syphilis. Tonsillitis. Tests for oxidizing enzymes to detect blood in stool or urine.

Side effects. Stomach inflammation. Intestinal pain. Diarrhea. Skin rashes.

Interactions. None reported.

Overdose. Intestinal pain. Nausea. Vomiting. Diarrhea.

Guarana Paullinia cupana, Brazilian Cocoa: contains caffeine, theobromine, theophylline, guaranine, guaranine

Uses. Arthritis. Astringent. Athletic performance. Bronchial constriction. Diarrhea. Diuretic. Fatigue.
Hangovers. Headaches. Impedes blood clots. Improve Promote memory. Increase metabolic rate. Obesity. Speed up digestive juices. Relax blood vessels. Heartbeat. Stimulate the CNS. Stimulate the urinary system. Strengthen heartbeat. Weight loss. Cardiovascular

Side effects. Anxiety. Cancer. Insomnia. disease. Decreased fertility. Hyperactivity. Take Panic. Palpitations. Trembling. Urinary frequency. Take care with heart conditions, high blood pressure,

Interactions. Caffeine and theophylline interact with other medications. Do not take with MAOIs or valium type medications. Do not take with heart medications. Do not take with caffeine. Do not take with birth control drugs. Do not take with Tagamet. Do not take with antibiotics. Do not take with Lithium.

Overdose. Abdominal spasms. Difficult urination. Vomiting.

Guggul Commiphora mukul, gugulipid, gum guggulu: contains guggulsterones, resin, volatile oils and gum.

Uses. Arthritis. Atherosclerosis. High cholesterol. High triglycerides. Obesity. Reduce the stickiness of platelets.

Side effects. Abdominal pain. Anorexia. Diarrhea. skin rash. Take care with liver disease, inflammatory bowel disease and diarrhea.

Interactions. Do not take with heart medication or aspirin.

Overdose. None reported. It would be reasonable to assume an exaggeration of side effects.

Gymnema Gymnema Gymnema sylvestre, gurmarbooti, periploca of the woods, meshasringi (ram's horn) : contains gymnemic acid, gurmarin, bymnemic acid

Uses. Adult-onset diabetes (NIDDM). Constipation. High cholesterol. High triglycerides. Liver disease. Stomach ailments. Water retention.

Side effects. None reported. If you have NIDDM do not treat yourself.

Interaction. None reported.

Overdose. None reported.

Haronga Haronga madagascariensis
Uses. Appetite loss. Dysentery. Indigestion. Kill certain bacteria. Protect liver.
Side Effects. Do not use with severe pancreas or liver disorder, gallstones, bile duct Obstruction, or other gallbladder problems. Sensitivity to light.
Interactions. None reported.
Overdose. None reported.

Hawthorn Crataegus laevigata, Crataegus oxyacantha, Crataegus monogyna, Whitethorn: contains bioflavonoids, oligomeric procyanidins, vitexin, quercetin and hyperoside, anthocyanin-type pigments, Cratagolic acid, Flavinonoid, Glycosides, Purines, Saponin
Uses. Angina pectoris. Antioxidant. Atherosclerosis. Congestive heart failure. High blood pressure. Improve blood flow to the heart muscle and extremities. Relax smooth muscle of uterus and intestines.
Side effects. Bronchial constriction. Depress respiration. Slow heart rate. Irregular heartbeats.
Interactions. Do not take if taking medicine for blood pressure or heart failure. Enhance effects of digitalis. Do not take with anesthesia.
Overdose. Breathing difficulties. Headache. Irregular heartbeat. Migraine. Nausea. Palpitations.

Heartsease Viola Tricolor, Johnny-jump-up, Wild Pansy
Uses. Constipation. Feverish colds. Poor metabolism. Respiratory and throat inflammation. Whooping cough. External. Acne. Cradle cap. Eczema. Female genital itching. Impetigo. Skin inflammation. Warts.

Side effects. None reported.
Interaction. None reported.
Overdose. Nausea. Vomiting.

Heather Celluna Vulgaris, Ling
Uses. Agitation. Cramps. Diarrhea. Digestive disorders. Improve bile flow. Inhibit bacteria. Insomnia. Kidneys and lower urinary tract. Bacteria and gallbladder disease. Prostate symptoms. Liver complaints. Rheumatism. Urinary problems. Respiratory wounds.
Side effects. None reported.
Interaction. None reported.
Overdose. None reported.

Heliotropium europaem Heliotrine Lassiocarpine
Uses. Improve bile production. Polyps. Tumors. Ulcers. Warts.
Side effects. Jaundice (yellow eyes and skin).
Overdose. Destroys liver cells.

Hellebore American Hellebore, Green Hellebore, Liliaceae: contains Veratrum viride, Germidine, Germitrine, Jervine, Pseudojervine, Rubijervine, veratrum, alkaloids
Uses. Depress central nervous system. High blood pressure. Slow heart rate. Toxemia of pregnancy.
Side effects. Abdominal pain. Burning sensation in mouth. Diarrhea. Headache. Irritate gastrointestinal system. Nausea.
Interactions. None reported.
Overdose. Sudden blood-pressure drop. Faintness. Cold sweat, Paleness. Rapid pulse. Vomiting.

Helonias False Unicorn Root, Fairy Wand, Chamaelirium lutem: contains Chamaelirin, saponin

Uses. Appetite loss. Astringent. Diuretic. Laxative. Prevents miscarriage.

Side effects. Diarrhea. Irritate gastrointestinal system. Nausea.

Interaction. None reported.

Hemp Nettle Galeopsis Segetum

Uses. Astringent. Bronchitis. Cough. Diuretic. Loosen phlegm. Lung conditions.

Side effects. None reported. Interactions. None reported.

Overdose. None reported.

Henbane Hyoscyamus niger, Devil's Eye, Hogbean, Poison Tobacco, Stinking Nightshade: contains hyoscyamine, scopolamine

Uses. Analgesia. Asthma. Epilepsy. Eye inflammation. Involuntary discharge of sperm. Liver and gallbladder problems. Meningitis. Mouthwash. Nervous conditions. Scabies. Scar tissue. Sedative. Stomach and intestinal cramps. Toothache. Tumors. Ulcers. Vaginal discharge. Whooping cough.

Side effects. Constipation. Dilated pupils. Dry mouth. Hallucinations. Impaired distance vision Increased heart rate. Reduced contractions of gastrointestinal tract. Reduced sweating. Urinary retention. Not for use with enlarged colon, fluid in the lungs, glaucoma, narrow stomach or intestinal passages, prostate cancer, rapid heartbeat.

Interactions. Can increase the severity of side effects of prescription drugs, including Amantadine (Symmetrel), Antihistamines, Antidepressants (tricyclic and MAO inhibitors i.e.

Elavil, Tofrani1-PM, Triavil, Nardil and Parnate, Parkinson's medication Elderpryl, Haloperidol (Ha Idol, and phenothiazines i.e. Compazine, Stelazine, and Thorazine, Procainamide (Procanbid) and Quinidine (Quinaglute, Quinidex).

Overdose. Delirium. Dry mouth. Enlarged pupils.
Fast, irregular heartbeat. Exhaustion and sleep Hallucinations. Hyperactivity. Suffocation. Reddened
Restlessness. Sleepiness. Death. skin.

Hibiscus Hibiscus sabdariffa, Guinea Sorrel, Jamaica Sorrel, Red Sorrel, Roselle
Uses. Appetite loss. Circulation disorders. Colds. constipation. Hypertension. Indigestion. Phlegm. Relax the uterus. Respiratory inflammation. Water retention. side effects. Laxative.
Interactions. None reported.
Overdose. None reported.

Hollyhock Alcea rosea, Althea Rose, Malva Flowers, Rose Mallow
Uses. Bronchitis. Cough. Fever. Indigestion. Kidney inflammation. Menstrual problems. Sore throat. External. Skin inflammation. Ulcers.
Side effects. None reported.
Interactions. None reported.
Overdose. None reported.

Hops Humulus lupulus: contains bitter substances, humulone and lupulone, 1-3% volatile oils, humulene, lupulinic acid, lupulon
Uses. Abrasions. Anti-inflammatory. Appetite stimulant. Bacteriostatic (inhibit to have a growth pillow filled with hops to encourage sleep) Depress central nervous system. Diuretic.

Dyspepsia. Flavoring agent in beer. Increase flow of digestive juices. Insomnia. Nervousness. Ulcers. Tonic. Treat sexual neuroses. External. Sores. Skin.

Side effects. Contact dermatitis. Hallucinations Avoid if depressed.

Interaction. Do not take with barbiturates, valium. type medications, sedating medications or alcohol.

Overdose. None reported.

Horehound Marrubium vulgare, Houndsbane: contains marrubiin, resin, tannins, volatile oils

Uses. Appetite loss. Asthma. Bronchitis. Cold. Constipation. Cough. Diarrhea. Expectorant. Gas. Increase perspiration. Indigestion. Jaundice. Liver and gallbladder problems. Loosen phlegm. Lung inflammation. Painful menstruation. Respiratory infections. Sores. Stimulate digestive juices. Stimulate production of bile. Thins mucus from lungs and bronchial tubes. Tuberculosis. Whooping cough. Liqueurs and aperitifs.

Side effects. Hypertension. Diarrhea. Nausea. Vomiting.

Interactions. May interfere with the absorption of vitamins, minerals or medications.

Overdose. None reported.

Horse chestnut Aesculus hippocastanum, Buckeye, Spanish Chestnut, Aesculin, argyroscin, capsuloescinic acid, escin, aescin: contains flavonoids, sterols and tannins.

Uses. Anti-inflammatory. Arthritis. Chronic venous insufficiency. Cough. Edema. Fever. Hemorrhoids. Improves the flow of blood to the heart • Increase bleeding time. Lower back pain. Nighttime cramps in the calves. Phlebitis. Premenstrual syndrome.

Rheumatism. Skin inflammation. Sprains. Varicose veins. Tones walls of the veins. External. Skin cancer. Skin ulcers.

Side effects. Avoid with liver or kidney disease. Irritation of the digestive tract. Kidney damage. Lack of coordination. Nausea. Unusual bleeding. Vomiting. External. Allergic Skin reactions.

Interactions. Do not take with blood thinners or aspirin.

Overdose. Diarrhea. Enlarge pupils. Loss consciousness. Reddening of the face. Severe thirst. Visual disturbance. Vomiting.

Horsemint Monarda punctata: contains carvacrol, d-limonene, hydrothymoquinone, linalool,
cyemene, monarda oil, thymol

Uses. Abdominal cramps. Gas. Kills intestinal parasites. Nausea. External. Antibacterial. Antifungal.

Side effects. Diarrhea. Irritates tissues and mucous membranes. Nausea. Skin rash. Vomiting.

Interactions. None reported.

Overdose. None reported. It would be reasonable to assume an exaggeration of side effects.

Horseradish Cochlearia armoracia, Armoracia nasticana, Armoraciae radix, Great Raifort, Mountain Radish, Red Cole: contains many compounds similar to
mustard, volatile oil, isothiocyanates, glycosides, allyl isothiocyanate, Sinigriu

Uses. Antibiotic. Bronchitis. Common cold. Cough. Digestive problems. Food. Gallbladder disorders. Gout. Indigestion. Medicine. Influenza. Liver disease. Rheumatism. Sinus congestion. Sore throat. Stomach cramps. External. Improves Urinary tract circulation when applied to the skin. Minor muscle

Restrains the growth of tumors. Used on arthritic Joints or irritated nerves.

Side effects. Diarrhea. Diarrhea with blood. Excessive sweating. Nausea. Vomiting. Vomiting with blood. Can irritate mucous membranes and stomach lining. Avoid with hypothyroid, kidney disease or ulcers. External. Skin reddening. Eye irritation and burning

Interactions. None reported

Overdose. None reported.

Horsetail Equisetum arvense, Shave grass, Scouring rush , Bottle -brush, Horse Willow, Paddock-pipes, Pewterwort, Toadpipe: contains silicic acid and silicates, provide approximately 2-3% elemental silicon, potassium, aluminum, manganese , aconitic acid, equisitine, fatty acids, nicotine, silica, starch

Uses. Arthritis. Anti-inflammatory. Bedwetting. Blood tonic. Brittle fingernails. Burns. Collagen. Diarrhea. Dyspepsia. Flush bacterial infections from the urinary tract. Fractures. Frostbite. Gout. Hair loss. Kidney and bladder stones. Menstrual bleeding. Nasal, pulmonary, and gastric bleeding. Osteoarthritis. Osteoporosis. Rheumatic diseases. Swelling. Tuberculosis. Urinary tract infections. Water retention. Wounds. External. Bleeding wounds. Eczema. Rapid healing. Strength connective tissue. Abrasive cleanser to scour pots or shave wood.

Side effects. Avoid with weak heart or kidney problems. Use with care with large area skin lesions

Interactions. Do not take with heart medications.

Overdose. Cold hands and feet. Fever. Gait disturbances. Heartbeat irregularities. Muscle weakness.
Weight loss. Use tinctures, fluid extracts or preparations that have been subjected to 100 degrees C.

Houseleek Jupiter's Eye, Thor's Beard, Sempervivum tectorum, Sempervivum: contains Malic acid

Uses. Astringent. Diuretic. Prevents secretions of fluids. External. Burns. Bruises. Insect bites. Skin disease.

Side effects. Vomiting. Watery, explosive diarrhea.

Interactions. None reported.

Overdose. None reported. It would be reasonable to assume an exaggeration of side effects.

Huckleberry Vaccinum myrtillus: contains fatty acids, hydroquinone, loeanolic acid, neomyrtillin, tannins, ursolic acid

Uses. Decrease blood sugar. Diarrhea. Diuretic. Gastroenteritis. Scurvy.

Side effects. Do not use if allergic to blueberries.

Interactions. May interfere with the absorption of vitamins, minerals or medications.

Overdose. None reported.

Hydrangea Seven Barks, Peegee, Hydrangea paniculata: contains hydrangin, resin, saponin, volatile oils

Uses. Astringent. Bladder stones. Cystitis. Dyspepsia. Gas. Prevent secretion of fluids.

Side effects. Hydrangin contains cyanide. Dizziness. Heavy feeling in chest. Nausea. Vomiting. Smoking: Hallucinations. Toxicity.

Interactions. None reported.

Overdose. None reported. It would be reasonable to assume an exaggeration of side effects.

Hyssop Hyssopus officinalis

Uses. Fevers. Gallbladder problems. Intestinal Respiratory ailments Liver complaints. Poor circulation.

Side effects. Long term use of oil may cause

Interaction. None reported.

Overdose. Seizures from oil.

Iceland Moss Etraria islandica, Eryngo-leaved Liverwort

Uses. Appetite loss. Bronchitis. Colds. Cough. Fever. Impaired immunity. Indigestion. Inflamed or irritated tissue. Kidney and bladder disorders. Lung disease. Poorly healing wounds. Sore throat.

Side effects. Sensitivity reactions.

Interactions. None reported.

Overdose. None reported.

Immortelle Helichrysum arenarium, Eternal Flower, Everlasting, Yellow Chaste Weed

Uses. Anti-bacterial. Appetite loss. Indigestion.
Liver and gallbladder problems. Promote bile production. Spasms. Water retention.

Side effects. Avoid or use with extreme caution with blocked bile duct or gallstones.

Interactions. None reported.

Overdose. None reported.

Indian Nettle Kuppi, Mercury Weed, Indian Acalypha, Hierba de Cancer, Acalypha indica, A. virginica: contains acalyphine, cyanogenic glycoside, inositol, methyl ether, resin, triacetomamine, volatile oils

Uses. Mouthwash. Laxative. Poultice. Thins mucus from lungs and bronchial tubes.

Side effects. Irritate stomach lining. Nausea. Vomiting. Diarrhea.

Interactions. None reported.

Overdose. None reported. It would be reasonable to assume an exaggeration of side effects.

Indian Tobacco Lobelia, Asthma Weed, Lobelia inflata: contains isolobenine, lobelanine, lobelidine, lobeline, nor-lobelaine

Uses. Asthma. Depress central nervous system (small amounts). Thins mucus from lungs and bronchial tubes. Weight loss. Stimulate central nervous system (large amounts) .

Side effects. Vomiting.

Interactions. None reported.

Overdose. Can be dangerous. Coma. Diarrhea. Excess salivation. Excess tear formation. Giddiness. Headache. Nausea. Stupor. Tremors. Vomiting.

Indigo Baptisia tinctoria: contains bapitoxine, baptisin, baptisine, cystisine, quinolizidine

Uses. Amebiasis. Anti-emetic. Antiseptic. Astringent. Colic. Colitis. Dysentery. Malaria. Nausea. Scarlet fever. Skin problems. Snakebite. Sores. Typhoid fever. Wounds.

Side effects. Irritate gastrointestinal lining membrane. Nausea. Vomiting. Diarrhea. Watery, explosive bowel movements.

Interactions. None reported.

Overdose. None reported. It would be reasonable to assume an exaggeration of side effects.

Iris Iris Species Orris Root

Uses. Bronchitis. Cough. Digestive problems.

Dysentery. Headaches. Jaundice. Pancreas conditions. Sore throat. Spitting up blood. Thyroid condition.

Side effects. Internal. Mucous membranes inflammation. Bloody diarrhea. Stomach pain. Vomiting. External. Irritation of skin and mucous membranes.

Interactions. None reported.

Overdose. None reported. It would be reasonable to assume an exaggeration of side effects.

Irish Moss Chondrus crispus, Gigartina calcium, carrageenan, chlorine contains bromine, protein, sodium

Uses. Abrasions. Cough. Constipation. Diarrhea. Gelatin in jelly. Hand lotion. Interferes with blood clotting mechanism.

Side effects. Nausea.

Interactions. Increase the effect of blood thinners. **Overdose**. None reported. It would be reasonable to assume an exaggeration of side effects.

Jambolan Syzygium cumini, Jambul, Jamum, Java plum, Rose Apple

Uses. Anti-inflammatory. Asthma. Astringent. Congestion. Diabetes. Diarrhea. Failing sexual desire.
Gargle. Gas. Indigestion. Mouth and throat inflammation. Skin ulcers. Sore throat. Spasms. Spleen problems. Stomach disorders. Water retention. Vaginal discharge. External. Superficial inflammation.

Side effects. None reported.

Interactions. None reported.

Overdose. None reported.

Japanese Mint Mentha arvensis, Var piperascens

Uses. Antibacterial. Bile production. Breathing problems. Bronchitis. Colds. Cooling effect. Cough. Decongestant. Fever. Gas. Headache. Heart problems • Improve immune system. Joint pain. Liver and gallbladder problems. Stimulate bile production. Pain. Sore throat • External. Muscle and nerve pain.

Side effects. Avoid with gallbladder problems' blocked bile ducts or liver damage. Stomach discomfort. Oil aggravates bronchial asthma.

Interactions. None reported.

Overdose. Can be fatal.

Java Tea Orthosiphon spicatus

Uses. Antiseptic. Diuretic. Gout. Kidney and bladder stones. Liver and gallbladder problems. smooth muscle spasms. Urinary tract infections Rheumatism.

Side effects. Do not use with poor heart or kidney function. Drink 2 quarts of liquid per day.

Interactions. None reported.

Overdose. None reported.

Javanese Tumeric Curcuma Xanthorrhizia

Uses. Appetite loss. Bloating. Discourage bile tumor growth. Increase production of bile. Indigestion. Liver and gallbladder problems.

Side effects. Avoid or use with caution with bile duct blockage or gallstones. Stomach problems.

Interactions. Do not take with blood thinners, Motrin type drugs or aspirin.

Overdose. Stomach problems.

Jimsonweed Datura stramonium, Apple of Peru, Devil's

Apple, Devil's Trumpet, Jamestown Weed, Mad-apple, Nightshade, Stinkweed, Thornapple

Uses. Asthma. Astringent. Bronchitis. Burns. Cough. Digestive system spasms. Parkinson's disease. Active ingredients in the prescription drugs Donnatal, Lomotil, and Urised.

Side effects. Avoid with glaucoma, obstruction irregular enlarged prostate,
heartbeat, swelling in lungs, difficulty passing urine, hardening of arteries. Plant is poisonous. Diminished Heat build-up because urination. Extreme constipation. Dry mouth.
of decreased perspiration. Skin reddening. Enlarged pupils. Fast, irregular heartbeat. Vision problems.

Interactions. None reported. Use is not recommended.

Overdose. Restlessness, compulsive speech, hallucinations, delirium, manic episodes, exhaustion, sleep respiratory failure and death.

Juniper Juniperus communis: contains volatile oils, particularly 4 -terpineol

Uses. Appetite loss. Belching. Bloating. Cancer. Diabetes. Diuretic. Flavoring agent in gin. Gout. Heartburn. Herpes simplex. High blood pressure. Indigestion. Kidney and bladder stones. Menstrual problems. Skin growths. Upset stomach. Urinary tract infections. Warts. External. Rheumatism.

Side effects. Do not take for more than six weeks. Do not take with kidney diseases or inflammation. Skin contact can cause a rash.

Interactions. None reported. Do not combine with diuretics.

Overdose. An overdose can damage the kidneys.

Kava Piper methysticum, Kava Kava: contains Kava-lactones called kava-pyrones

Uses. Anxiety. Heighten sensory perception. Improve mental acuity. Insomnia. Mellowing effects. Memory. Nervousness. Pain. Produces state of contentment. Provides feeling of well-being.

Side effects. Allergic skin rash. Depression; avoid with history of depression. Mild gastrointestinal upset. Initially may cause feeling tired upon awakening. visual disturbances.

Interactions. Do not take with alcohol, barbiturates benzodiazepams, antidepressants, antipsychotic drugs' or sedating drugs. Do not take with drugs for Parkinson's

Overdose. Difficulty focusing. Gastrointestinal complaints. Lack of coordination. Loss of balance. May turn skin yellow temporarily. Pupil dilation. Tiredness. Tendency to sleep.

Khella Ammi visnaga

Uses. Abdominal cramps. Asthma. Bronchitis. Chest pain (angina). Cough. High blood pressure. Improve pumping action of heart. Irregular heartbeat. Kidney stones. Liver and gallbladder problems. Smooth muscle spasms (airways, blood vessels, tubes and ducts). Whooping cough. External. Inflammation. Poisonous bites. Wounds.

Side effects. Dizziness. Headache. Jaundice. Loss of appetite. Nausea. Sensitivity to sunlight. Sleep disorders.

Interactions. None reported.

Overdose. It would be reasonable to assume an exaggeration of side effects. Liver problems.

Knotweed Polygonum aviculare, Allseed, Nine-joints, Armstrong, Beggarweed, Bird's Tongue , Birdweed, Centinode, Cow Grass, Crawlgrass, Doorweed, Hogweed, Knotgrass, Pigweed, Red Robin, Sparrow Tongue, Swine's Grass

Uses. Astringent. Bronchitis. Cough. Decreases

perspiration. Dysentery. Gonorrhea. Hemorrhage. Improves urination. Itching. Jaundice. Lung problems. Sore throat. External uses. Various skin disorders.

Side effects. None reported.

Interactions. None reported.

Overdose. None reported.

Kudzu Pueraria lobata, common name Ge-gen, Peuraria thomsonii: contains isoflavones, daidzin, puerarin and daidzein

Uses. Alcoholism. Allergies. Arteriosclerosis. Circulation to heart muscle. Diarrhea. High blood pressure. Measles. Migraine. Thirst. Headache. Stiff neck with pain combination.

Side effects. None reported.

Interactions. None reported.

Overdose. None reported.

Lady's Mantle Alchemilla vulgaris, Bear' s Foot, Lion's Foot, Nine Hooks, Stellaria

Uses. Astringent. Diarrhea. Eczema. Inhibit pancreatic enzyme production. Menopause. Menstrual pain. Mouth and throat infections. Skin rashes. Stomach Problems.

Side effects. None reported. If it inhibits pancreatic enzyme production, take with caution if you have a disorder of the pancreas.

Interactions. None reported. May interfere with medications for the pancreas.

Overdose. None reported.

Laminaria Laminaria hyperborean

Uses. Thyroid problems

Side effects. Severe allergic reaction. Can create or exacerbate overactive thyroid.

Interactions. None reported. May increase action of thyroid supplements.

Overdose. Agitation. Fatigue. Insomnia. Increased appetite. Increased sweating. Nervousness. Palpitations. Rapid heartbeat. Thyroid enlargement. Weakness. Weight loss.

Larch Latrix decidua
Uses. Blood pressure. Bronchitis. Colds. Cough. Fever. Improve immune system. Rheumatism. Sore throat.
Side effects. Inhaling can aggravate throat and lungs.
Interactions. None reported.
Overdose. External. Has potential to damage kidneys or nervous system.

Lavender Lavandula Angustifolia
Uses. Abdominal problems. Appetite. Gas. Improve bile production. Insomnia. Mood disorders. Nervousness. Sedative. External uses. Bath additive. Improve circulation. Fragrance. Spike Lavender acts as insect repellent.
Side effects. Allergy to oil.
Interactions. None reported.
Overdose. None reported.

Lemon balm Melissa official is, Balm Mint, Bee Balm, Blue Balm, Cure-all, Garden Balm, Honey Plant, Sweet Balm, Sweet Mary: contains terpenes, flavonoids, polyphenolics, and other compounds
Uses. Antibacterial. Antihistamine. Anti-inflammatory. Antiseptic. Antispasmodic. Antiviral. Asthma. Bloating. Bronchitis. Colic. Depression. Diarrhea. Dizziness. Earache. Fever. Gas. Graves disease. Headache. Herpes simplex. High blood pressure. Indigestion.

Memory loss. Nausea. Nervousness. Palpitations. Sedative. Toothache. Vomiting. External. To temples for insomnia or nerve pain.

Side effects. Avoid with glaucoma, may raise pressure in the eye.

Interactions. Do not take with heart medications. Do not take with thyroid medications. Do not take with diuretics. Do not take with antacids.

Overdose. None reported.

Lemongrass Cymbopogen citratus
Uses. Acne. Analgesic. Antiseptic. Athletes foot. Diarrhea. Fever. Flu. Headache. Sedative. Stomachache
Side effects. None reported.
Interactions. None reported.
Overdose. None reported.

Licorice Glycyrrhiza glabra, Glycyrrhiza uralensis: contains glycyrrhizin, flavonoids
Uses. Addison's disease. Anti-inflammatory. Antioxidants. Antiviral. Asthma. Boils. Bronchitis. Canker sores (mouth ulcers). Chronic fatigue syndrome. Coughs. Decongestant. Demulcent for digestive and urinary tracts (soothing, coating). Diabetes. Eczema. Excessive thirst. Fibromyalgia. Flavoring. Headache. Heartburn. Herpes simplex. Indigestion. Inhibits the breakdown of the cortisol produced by the body. Peptic ulcer. Protect liver cells. Sore throats. Stomach inflammation. Tuberculosis.
Side effects. Increase blood pressure. Water retention. Aggravates chronic hepatitis, cirrhosis of the liver, or slowed flow of bile from the liver. Avoid with abnormal muscle tension, poor kidney

function, or low potassium levels. Take licorice preparations without the glycyrrhizin (deglycyrrhizinated).

Interactions e Increase potassium loss used with drugs, like Diuril, Zaroxolyn, and others. Increase effects of drugs with digitalis- like compounds, i.e. Lanoxin. Increase effects and side effects of steroid type medications, i.e. prednisone. Do not take with heart medications, blood pressure medications, diuretics or steroids.

Overdose. High doses can lead to excessive loss salt from the blood, water retention, high blood pressure, and heart irregularities.

Lily of the Valley Convallaria majalis, Jacob's Ladder, May Bells, May Lily

Uses. Circulation problems. Conjunctivitis ("pinkeye"). Epilepsy. High blood pressure. Improve labor contractions. Irregular heartbeat. Kidney and bladder stones. Leprosy. Palpitations. Paralysis. Strokes. Swelling. Urinary tract infections. Weak heart.

Side effects. Nausea. Vomiting. Headache. Irregular heartbeat. Stupor. Visual disturbances.

Interactions. Calcium. Laxatives. Quinidine. Quinaglute. Quinidex. Hydrocortisone. Prednisone. Lasix. HydroDIURIL.

Overdose. Potentially fatal disruptions of heartbeat.

Linden Tilia species, Common Lime, European Lime
Uses. Bronchitis. Cough. Cramps. Diuretic. Enhance sweating. Irritation. Loosen phlegm. Nerves. Stomach problems.

Side effects. None reported.
Interactions. None reported.
Overdose. None reported.

Linseed Linum usitatissimum, Flax: contains prussic acid

Uses. Chest congestion. Constipation. Diarrhea. Gonorrhea. Irritated bladder. Irritated gastrointestinal tract. Irritated throat. Laxative. Lung problems. Prevent cancer. Reduce fat. Reduce sugar. External. Combine with limewater for skin inflammation, burns and scalds

Side effects. Avoid with bowel obstruction, narrowed digestive tract, or severe inflammation of gastrointestinal tract.

Interactions. None reported. May interfere with the absorption of vitamins, minerals and medications.

Overdose. Can lead to bowel obstruction if not taken with enough fluid. Poisoning.

Lovage Levisticum officinale, Sea Parsley

Uses. Antiseptic. Diuretic. Gas. Heartburn. Indigestion. Kidney and bladder stones. Menstrual problems. Respiratory inflammation. Sedative. Spasms of smooth muscles. Stimulate digestive juices. Urinary tract infections.

Side effects. Avoid if water retention is from a weak heart or kidneys. Avoid with inflammation in the urinary system. Increased sensitivity to sun.

Interactions. None reported.

Overdose. None reported.

Luffa Luffa aegyptica

Uses. Colds. Lowered resistance. Sinus inflammation. Bath sponge (loofah). Baskets. Shoe soles. Oil filters. Sound-deadening construction material.

Side effects. None reported.

Interactions. None reported.

Overdose. None reported.

Lungwort Pulmonaria officinalis, Dage of Jerusalem
Uses. Bronchitis. Cough. Diuretic. Mild upper respiratory problems. External. Astringent. Treat
wounds.
Side effects. None reported.
Interactions. None reported.
Overdose. None reported.

Lycium Lycium barbarum, Lycium chinense, Chinese Wolfberry
Uses. Berries. Blurred eyesight. Circulation. Dizziness. Protect liver and kidneys from toxins. Ringing in the ears. Vision problems. Root. Cough. Fever. High blood pressure. Stimulate the nervous system of the internal organs. Wheezing.
Side effects. Worsen inflammation. Aggravate poor digestion. Increase bloating.
Interactions. None reported.
Overdose. None reported.

Magnolia Flower Magnolia Liliflora, Xin yi hua
Uses. Asthma. Congestion. Consumption. Cough. Cramps. Diarrhea. Fungicide. Malaria. Muscle relaxant. Nausea. Nervous stomach. Parasite. Rheumatism. Sores. Toothache. Used for quinine. Vomiting. Wounds. Combined with angelica, mint and chrysanthemum for upper respiratory tract infections. External. Astringent.
Side effects. Hairy outer layer of buds can irritate, remove it.
Interactions. None reported.
Overdose. Dizziness. Red eyes.

Maidenhair Adiantum capillus-veneris, Five-finger

93

Fern, Hair of Venus, Maiden Fern, Rock Fern

Uses. Asthma. Bites. Bronchitis. Chills. Congestion. Cough. Fever. Heart trouble. Menstrual difficulties. Respiratory tract problems. External. Healthy skin tone. Impetigo. Rinse for dandruff and thinning hair. Stings.

Side effects. None reported.
Interactions. None reported.
Overdose. None reported.

Maitake Grifola Frondosa, Dancing Mushroom: beta-D-glucan
Uses. Cancer. Chemotherapy support. Diabetes. High cholesterol. High triglycerides. HIV support. Hypertension. Immune function. Tonic. Obesity. Boost wellness and vitality.

Side effects. None reported.
Interactions. None reported.
Overdose. None reported.

Male Fern Dryopteris filix-mas, Aspidium, Bear's Paw Root, Knotty Brake, Sweet Brake
Uses. Anti-viral. Lymph system problems. Worms. External. Earache. Muscle pain. Nerve pain. Rheumatism. Sciatica. Sleeplessness. Teething. Toothache. As smoke. Snakes. Gnats.

Side effects. Diarrhea. Nausea. Queasiness. Severe headache. Vomiting. Do not use if elderly, anemic, diabetic, or have a heart condition, kidney problems, or liver disease.

Interactions. None reported.
Overdose. Blindness. Heart, kidney and liver damage. Mental disorders. Paralysis. Spasms. Visual damage. Death.

Manna Fraxinus ornus, Flowering Ash

Uses. Constipation. Fissures. Hemorrhoids. Rectal surgery. Softens stool.

Side effects. Avoid with intestinal obstruction. Nausea. Gas.

Interactions. None reported.

Overdose. None reported. It would be reasonable to assume an exaggeration of side effects.

Marigold Calendula officinalis

Uses. Calm central nervous system. Constipation. Convulsions. Diuretic. Eye inflammation. Fever. Heart stimulant. Improve bile production. Improve immune system. Inflammation. Liver disease. Menstrual cramps. Slows tumor growth. Sore throat. Stomach ulcers. Tired limbs. Toothache. Worms. External. Acne. Antifungal. Antimicrobial. Antiviral. Bee stings. Blood clots in the veins. Boils. Burns. Chronic skin inflammation. Clean wounds. Cosmetics. Dry skin. Eczema. Frostbite. Improves wound healing. Inflamed veins. Rectal and anal inflammation. Skin preparations. Treat enlarged and flamed lymph glands. Varicose veins.

Side effects. Increased sensitivity.

Interactions. None reported.

Overdose. None reported. It would be reasonable to assume an exaggeration of side effects

Marjoram Origanum majorana

Uses. Antiseptic. Common cold. Cough. Dizziness. Headache. Nervous conditions. Stomach pain.

Side effects. None reported.

Interactions. None reported.

Overdose. None reported.

Marshmallow Althea officinalis, Cheeses, Mallards, Mortification Root, Schloss Tea, Sweet Weed, Wymote: contains large carbohydrate (sugar) molecules, mucilage

Uses. Anti-infective. Asthma. Bronchitis. Burns. Chron's disease. Colds. Constipation. Cough. Diarrhea. Improve immune system. Increase production of white blood cells. Infected wounds. Inflamed mucus membranes. Reduce sugar level in body. Slow mucus production. Sore mouth. Sore throat. Ulcers.

Side effects. None reported. Syrup is concentrated sugar.

Interactions. May interfere with the absorption of vitamins, minerals and medications.

Overdose. None reported.

Mate Ilex paraguariensis, Jesuit's Tea, Paraguay Tea, Yerba Mate

Uses. Diuretic. Fatigue. Heart palpitations. Improve force of heartbeat. Irregular heartbeat. Kidney and bladder stones. Metabolizes sugars and fats. Stimulate central nervous system. Urinary tract infections.

Side effects. Diarrhea. Dizziness. Headache. Insomnia. Irregular heart rhythm. Irritability. Loss of appetite. Palpitations. Restlessness. Vomiting. Do not take if sensitive to caffeine.

Interactions. None reported.

Overdose. Heart irregularities. Muscle spasms. Stiffness.

Meadowsweet Filipendula ulmaria, Bridewort, Meadow-wort, Queen of the Meadow, Spireaea ulmaria

Uses. Astringent. Bronchitis. Cough. Diuretic. Flu. Gout. Inflammation. Kidney and bladder inflammation. Rheumatism.

Side effects. Avoid if sensitive to aspirin (salicylate).

Interactions. Do not take if on blood thinners or aspirin.
Overdose. Queasiness. Stomach problems.

Melatonin
Uses. Aging. Alzheimer's. Cancer. Cholesterol. High blood pressure. Insomnia. Jet lag. Promote normal sleep. Regulate body rhythms. Seasonal affective disorder (SAD).

Side effects. Disrupted sleep patterns. Headache. Rash. Upset stomach. Avoid with AIDS, autoimmune disease, rheumatoid arthritis, depression, diabetes, emotional disorder, epilepsy, heart disease, leukemia, lymph system disorders, multiple sclerosis, osteoarthritis, or serious allergies . If attempting to conceive avoid this hormone. Do not drive or operate machinery.

Interactions. Beta blockers such as Inderal, Lopressor, and Tenormin. Large amounts of ibuprofen (Motrin, Advil) . Mood-altering drugs i.e. diazepam
(Valium). Steroid medications i.e. prednisone.

Overdose. None reported. It would be reasonable to assume an exaggeration of side effects.

Milk Thistle Silybum marianum, Our Lady's Thistle: contains bioflavonoid complex, silymarin, silibinin, silidianin, silicristin.

Uses. Antidote for death-cap mushroom poisoning. Antioxidant. Appetite loss. Cirrhosis. Eradicate free radicals. Gallbladder problems. Hepatitis. Inflammatory liver disease. Jaundice. Liver damage. Obstructions of spleen. Promote growth of new liver cells. Psoriasis.
Relieve liver, spleen or kidney congestion.
Side effects. Laxative.

Interactions. None reported. May interfere with the absorption of vitamins, minerals and medications.
Overdose. None reported.

 Milkweed Asclepias
 Uses. Anti-inflammatory. Antiseptic. Asthma. Bronchitis. Diaphoretic (promotes perspiration).
Diarrhea. Diuretic. Emetic. Expectorant. Fever. Heart trouble. Intestinal problems. Pleurisy. Pneumonia.
Rheumatism. Snakebite. Stomach problems. Warts.
 Side effects. None reported.
 Interactions. None reported.
 Overdose. Poisoning. No signs listed.

 Mint Mentha, Pennyroyal
 Uses. Colic. Cough. Croup. Diaphoretic (promotes perspiration). Digestion. Fever. Gas. Headache
Menstrual pain. Nausea. Nerves. Pneumonia. Rheumatism. Scabies. Sore muscles. Sore throat. Virus. External. Insect repellent.
 Side effects. Irritate mucous membranes. Reduce milk flow.
 Interactions. None reported.
 Overdose. Abortion. Coma. Convulsions. Severe liver damage.

 Mistletoe Viscum album, All-heal, Birdlime, Devil's fuge, Mystyldene
 Uses. Arteriosclerosis. Asthma. Chorea (rapid, jerky movements). Convulsions. Diarrhea. Dizziness. Exhaustion. Gout. Hysteria. Improve circulation. Internal bleeding. Loss of menstrual cycle. Low blood pressure. Rapid heartbeat. Relaxation of tight muscles. Rheumatism. Symptoms of malignant tumors. Tranquilizer. Tumor. Whooping cough.

Side effects. Allergic reactions. Chest pain (angina). Chills. Fever. Headache. Low blood pressure. Injections are not recommended for chronic infection,
i.e. allergic tendencies, or high fever. May cause local skin reactions, i.e. swelling and dead skin.

Interactions. None reported.

Overdose. None reported. It would be reasonable to assume an exaggeration of side effects

Motherswort Leonurus cardiaca, Lion's Ear, Lion's Tail, Throw-wort

Uses. Gas. Hyperthyroid. Irregular heartbeat Relaxing effect on the heart. Sedative. Weak heart.

Side effects. Do not take with a heart condition.

Interactions. Do not take with Tegretol or Tetracycline. Do not take with barbiturates, valium-type medications or alcohol.

Overdose. None reported.

Mountain Ash Berry Sorbus aucuparia, Rowan Tree, Sorb Apple, Witchen

Uses. Constipation. Diabetes. Diarrhea. Excess acid in the blood. Gout. Internal inflammations. Kidney disease. Lung infections. Menstrual difficulties. Poor metabolism. Rheumatism. Sinus and throat inflammations. Vitamin C deficiency. Used in marmalades, jams, jellies, fruit sauces, liqueur, and vinegar.

Side effects. Fresh berries. Stomach pain. uneasiness. Vomiting. Diarrhea. Kidney damage. Skin rashes. Drying or cooking berries reduces this effect.

Interactions. None reported.

Overdose. None reported. It would be reasonable to assume an exaggeration of side effects.

Mountain Flax Linum catharticum, Dwarf Flax, Fairy Flax, Mill Mountain, Purging Flax

Uses. Constipation. Cough. Edema. Hemorrhoids. Induce vomiting. Internal inflammation. Rheumatic disorders. Worms.

Side effects. Diarrhea. Inflammation of digestive system. Vomiting.

Interactions. None reported.

Overdose. Death.

Mugwort Common Wormwood, Felon Herb, St. John's Plant

Uses. Antimicrobial. Anxiety. Convulsions. Depression. Fatigue. Indigestion. Insomnia. Poor circulation. Protection from evil spirits. Restlessness. Stomachache. Sunstroke. Worms. Vomiting.

Side effects. Allergic skin reaction.

Interactions. None reported.

Overdose. None reported. It would be reasonable to assume an exaggeration of side effects.

Muira-Puama Ptychopetalum olacoides

Uses. Impotence.

Side effects. None reported.

Interactions. None reported.

Overdose. None reported.

Mullein Verbascum thapsus, Verbascum densiflorum, Aaron's Rod, Adam's Flannel, Beggar's Blanket, Feltwort, Golden Rod, Jacob's Staff, Shepherd's Club, Torchweed, Velvet Plant: mucilage, saponins, tannins.

Uses. Anticoagulant. Asthma. Bronchitis. Common cold. Convulsions. Cough. Cramps. Demulcent. Edema. Expectorant. Gout. Piles. Pneumonia. Recurrent ear infections. Rheumatism. Sore throat. Wounds. External. Inflammatory skin conditions. Burns. Insecticide. Irritated mucous membranes.

Side effects. Skin irritation.

Interactions. None reported. If leaves contain anticoagulant, avoid with blood thinners.

Overdose. None reported. It would be reasonable to assume an exaggeration of side effects.

Mustard Sinapis alba, White mustard

Uses. Antibacterial. Asthma. Bronchitis. Colds. Congestion. Constipation. Cough. Dropsy. Fever. Flushed skin. Improve immune system. Indigestion. Paralysis. Rheumatism. Sore throat. Sore muscles. Toothache.

Side effects. Inflammatory Kidney disease. Irritate internal membranes. Nerve damage. Stomach disorders. Stomach ulcers. External. Skin injury.

Interactions. None

Overdose. None reported. It would be reasonable to assume an exaggeration of side effects.

Myrrh Commiphora molmol: contains resin, gum, volatile iol

Uses. Analgesic. Antimicrobial. Astringent. Athletes foot. Bad breath. Bleeding disorders. Cancer. Canker sores (mouth ulcers). Common cold. Dental conditions. Disinfectant. Gas. Gingivitis (periodontal disease). Indigestion. Leprosy. Loosen phlegm. Missed menstrual periods. Poor circulation. Skin diseases. Sore throat. Stimulate macrophages (a type of white blood cell). Stomach pain. Syphilis. Wounds.

Side effects. None reported.

Interactions. None reported. If Myrrh helps with bleeding disorders, it would be reasonable to assume it would interfere with blood thinners.

Overdose. None reported.

Nasturtium Tropaeolum majus, Indian Cress

Uses. Antibacterial. Antifungal. Bronchitis. Cough. Urinary tract infections. External. Improve circulation.

Side effects. Irritate gastrointestinal lining. Irritate skin. Irritate stomach. Avoid with kidney disease.

Interactions. None reported.

Overdose. None reported. It would be reasonable to assume an exaggeration of side effects.

Nettle Urtica dioica: contains polysaccharides (complex sugars), lectins (large protein-sugar combination molecules)

Uses. Anti-inflammatory. Arthritis. BPH (benign prostate hypertrophy). Cloth. Cough. Food source. Hair growth. Hay fever. Pregnancy. Tuberculosis.

Side effects. Skin rash from contact.

Interactions. None reported.

Overdose. None reported.

Niauli Melaleucea viridiflora

Uses. Bactericidal. Bronchitis. Cough. Improves circulation.

Side effects. Nausea. Vomiting. Diarrhea. Avoid with liver disease, stomach inflammation, intestinal inflammation, or gallbladder disease. External. To the face can cause throat spasms, asthma-like attacks, and asphyxiation.

Interactions. Increases liver' s processing of medications, giving them less time in the body and by that action may decrease the effects of many drugs.

Overdose. Drop in blood pressure. Circulation problems. Collapse. Asphyxiation.

Nightshade Solanum dulcamara, Bittersweet, Felonwood, Fever Twig, Staff Vine

Uses. Antibacterial. Antispasmodic. Astringent. Anti-inflammatory. Blood purification. Boils. Eczema. Eye irritation. Fever. Insomnia. Parasites. Rabies. Skin conditions. Tuberculosis. Warts.

Side effects. Poisoning.

Interactions. None reported.

Overdose. Nausea. Vomiting. Enlarged pupils. Diarrhea. Death.

Notoginseng Root Panax notoginseng, San Qi, Pseudoginseng Root

Uses. Angina. Arteriosclerosis. Chron i s disease. High blood pressure. Internal bleeding. Speeds clotting. External. Anti-inflammatory.

Side effects. None reported.

Interactions. None reported. If speeds clotting, may interfere with blood thinners.

Overdose. None reported.

Nutmeg Myristica fragrans, Mace

Uses. Abdominal pain. Diarrhea. Flavoring. Impotence. Indigestion. Inflammation. Liver disease. Vomiting.

Side effects. External. Allergic skin reaction.

Interactions. None reported. Not recommended for medicinal use.

Overdose. Thirst. Nausea. Reddening and swelling of the face. Feeling of urgency. Altered consciousness. Hallucinations. Palpitations. Seizures. Shock.

Oats Aven sative, Groats, Oatmeal: contains alkaloids gramine and avenine, saponins avenacosides A and B, iron, manganese, zinc, silica

Uses. Anti-inflammatory. Anxiety. Bladder disorders. Boils. Cold gores. Depression. Diarrhea. Eczema. Edema. Flu. Fractures. High cholesterol. High triglycerides. Insomnia Nervous exhaustion. Nicotine withdrawal. Rheumatic condition. Sedative. Sore throat. External. Chronically cold or tired feet. Eye problems. Frostbite. Gout Impetigo (a contagious skin eruption. Itching. Skin Irritating.

Side effects. None reported. Avoid with celiac disease (gluten sensitivity)

Interactions. None reported.

Overdone. None reported.

Oleander Nerium odoratum, Rose Laurel

Uses. Heart failure. Hemorrhoids. Improve force of heartbeat. Nervous conditions. Scabies. Slow heart rate.

Side effects. Nausea. Vomiting. Diarrhea. Headache. Stupor. Irregular heartbeat.

Interactions. Increase effects of calcium salts, digitalis-type medications i.e. Lanoxin, diuretics, laxatives, Quinidine i.e. Quinaglute, Quinidex.

Overdose. Irregular heartbeat. Death.

Olive Leaf Olea europaea

Uses. High blood pressure. Liver and gallbladder problems. Regulate heartbeat. Spasms.

    Side effects. Aggravate gallstone problems.

    Interactions. None reported.

    Overdose. None reported.

Onion Allium cepa

    Uses. Antibacterial. Appetite loss. Arteriosclerosis. Asthma. Bronchitis. Chest pain (angina). Colds. Cough. Dehydration. Diabetes. Fever. Gallbladder problems. High blood pressure. Improve immune system. Indigestion.

Lower cholesterol. Menstrual problems. Parasite. Prevent clots. Sore throat. Thin blood. Whooping cough. External. Boils. Bruises. Burns. Insect bites. Warts. Wounds.

    Side effects. Stomach problems. External. Rash.

    Interactions. None reported. If thins blood it is reasonable to assume it will increase actions of blood thinners.

    Overdose. None reported.

Oregano Origanum vulgare, Mountain Mint, Wild Marjoram, Winter Marjoram, Wintersweet: contains thymol, carvacrol

    Uses. Bloating. Bronchial spasms. Bronchitis. Coughs. Diarrhea. Expectorant. Fever. Gas. Itchy skin. Jaundice. Lack of perspiration. Painful menstruation. Respiratory problems. Rheumatoid arthritis. Swollen glands. Urinary tract problems. Vomiting. External. Sores and aching muscles.

    Side effects. None reported.

    Interactions. None reported.

    Overdose. None reported.

Papaya Carica papaya, Melon Tree, Papaw: contains papain

Uses. Constipation. Digestive disorders. Leprosy. Worms. External. Cleans dead tissue from wounds.

Side effects. Allergic reactions. Aggravate bleeding disorders.

Interactions. Do not take with blood thinners or aspirin.

Overdose. None reported.

Parsley Petroselinum crispum

Uses. Edema. Failure to menstruate. Food. Jaundice. Kidney and bladder stones. Stomach and intestinal disorders. Urinary tract infections. Trigger and strengthen contractions of the uterus. External. Insect bites.

Side effects. Abortion. Allergic reactions. reaction. Sun sensitivity. Avoid with heart or kidney condition or kidney inflammation.

Interactions. Do not take with Tegretol or Tetracycline.

Overdose. Contractions of the bladder, intestines and uterus. Excessive weight loss, bloody stools, nosebleeds, and kidney failure.

Passion Flower Passiflora incarnata, Granadilla, Maypop, Passion Vine: contains harmane alkaloids, flavonoids

Uses. Anxiety. Asthma. Bladder problems. Boils. Chest complaints. Connective tissue disorders. Constipation. Depression. Diabetes. Diarrhea. Digestive problems. Epilepsy. Fatigue. Gallbladder complaints. Gastrointestinal spasms. Gout. Heart disease. Insomnia. Kidney disorders. Morning sickness. Muscle relaxant. Narcotic withdrawal. Nerve disorders. Nervous restlessness. Neuralgia. Overwork. Rheumatism. Sedative. Stress. Throat complaints. Tobacco withdrawal. Whooping cough. Worry. External. Antiseptic. Hemorrhoids. Wounds.

Side effects. Drowsiness.

Interactions. Avoid with MAO inhibiting antidepressant drugs. Do not take with barbiturates, valium- type medications, sedating drugs or alcohol.

Overdose. None reported.

Pau D'Arco Tabebuia impestiginosa, lapacho, taheebo, Trumpet Tree: contains lapachol, beta-lapachone, naphthaquinones

Uses. Antibacterial. Antifungal. Anti- inflammatory. Antiviral. Backache. Cancer. Diabetes. Hodgkins. Infectious diseases. Low sexual drive. Lupus. Parasites. Sexually transmitted diseases. Toothache. Wounds. Yeast infection.

Side effects. Uncontrolled bleeding. Nausea. Vomiting.

Interactions. If taken with other herbs, reduce dose. Do not take with blood thinners or aspirin.

Overdose. Uncontrolled bleeding. Nausea. Vomiting.

Pennyroyal Mentha pulegium, Lurk-in-the-Ditch, Mosquito Plant, Piliolerial, Pudding Grass, Run-by-the-Ground, Squaw Balm, Squawmint, Tickweed

Uses. Colds. Cramps. Excessive urination. Gout. Indigestion. Liver and gallbladder complaints. Respiratory problems. Skin inflammations.

Side effects. Abortion. Toxic to liver. Dried herb may be taken internally. Oil for external use.

Interactions. None reported.

Overdose. Vomiting. High blood pressure. Paralysis. Death from respiratory failure.

Peony Paeonia officinalis

Uses. Allergies. Chronic weakness. Disorders of mucous membranes. Epilepsy. Excitability. Fatigue. Gout. Hemorrhoids.

Improve muscular tension. Menstrual disorders. Migraine. Nerve pain. Respiratory problems. Rheumatism. Skin diseases. Ulcers. Whooping cough.

Side effects. Abortion. Cramps. Diarrhea. Stomach complaints. Vomiting.

Interactions. None reported.

Overdose. Cramps. Diarrhea. Vomiting.

Peppermint Mentha piperita, Brandy Mint, Black mint, White mint: contains volatile oil, free menthol, menthol. Lamb Mint is a hybrid of water mint and spearmint.

Uses. Appetite loss. Bronchitis. Colds. Cough. Decongestant. Digestive aid. Digestive cramps. Fever. Gingivitis (periodontal disease). Headache (tension). Improve immune system. Indigestion. Intestinal colic. Irritable bowel syndrome. Liver and gallbladder problems. Morning sickness. Nausea. Painful menstruation. Sore throat. Vomiting. Found in over the counter cough drops. External. Analgesic. Cooling effect on skin. Counterirritant. Improve blood flow to the affected area. Found in over the counter medicated rubs.

Side effects. Allergic reactions. Burning stomach upset. Avoid with acid reflux, chronic heartburn, blocked bile ducts, gallbladder inflammation, liver damage. Applied to face can created asthma-like symptoms or respiratory failure.

Interactions. None reported.

Overdose. Pure menthol can be fatal.

Periwinkle Vinca minor, Myrtle

Uses. Astringent. Brain hemorrhages. Circulatory problems. Diarrhea. Headache. Hemorrhoids. High blood pressure. Nosebleed. Skin conditions. Sore throat. Toothache. Wounds.

Side effects. Reddened skin. Stomach problems.

Interactions. None reported.

Overdose. Poisoning. Severe drop in blood pressure. Madagascar periwinkle is poisonous.

Balsam of Peru Myroxylon balsamum, Balsam of Tolu, Balsam Tree

Uses. Bronchitis. Colds. Cough. Expectorant. Fever. Hemorrhoids. Improve immune system. Sore throat. External. Antibacterial. Bedsores. Bruises caused by artificial limbs. Burns. Frostbite. Hemorrhoids. Infected wounds. Kills parasites, i.e. scabies. Leg ulcers. Poorly healing wounds. Wounds.

Side effects. Allergic reactions. Kidney damage kidneys. External. Skin reactions, i.e. eruptions, ulcers, swelling, and red patches. Sun sensitivity.

Interactions. None reported.

Overdose. None reported. It would be reasonable to assume an exaggeration of side effects.

Petasite Petasites hybridus, Blatterdock, Bog Rhubarb, Butterbur, Flapperdock, Langwort, Umbrella Leaves

Uses. Abdominal cramps. Appetite stimulant. Asthma. Breathing problems. Cough. Gallbladder problems. Headache. Kidney and bladder stones. Liver problems.
Pancreas. Restlessness. Sleep. Whooping cough. External. Malignant ulcers. Wounds.

Side effects. Birth defects. Cancer. Genetic damage. Liver damage. Take purified preparations with minimal pyrrolizidine.

Interactions. None reported.

Overdose. None reported.

Phyllanthus Phyllanthus niruri, Bahupatra, bhuiamla:

contains lignans, phyllanthine, hypophyllanthine, alkaloids, bioflavonoids, quercetin.

Uses. Diabetes. Frequent menstruation. Gonorrhea. Hepatitis B. Jaundice. Liver disorders. External. Itchiness. Skin ulcers. Sores. Swelling.

Side effects. None reported.

Interactions. None reported.

Overdose. None reported.

Pilewort Ranunculus ficaria, Figwort, Lesser Celandine, Smallwort

Uses. Bleeding gums. Burns. Swollen joints. Vitamin C deficiency (scurvy). Wounds. External. Hemorrhoids. Scratches. Warts. Wounds.

Side effects. Abdominal pain. Diarrhea. Irritation of intestines. Irritation of urinary tract. Rapid Heartbeat. Stomach irritation. External. Blisters. Burns.

Interactions. None reported.

Overdose. Fresh picked Pilewort. Asphyxiation. Dried is relatively safe.

Pimpinella Pimpinella Major, Burnet Saxifrage, Lesser Burnet, Pimpernella

Uses. Bronchitis. Cough. Decongestant. Decreases bronchial secretions. Digestive stimulant. Upper respiratory irritation. Urinary problems. External. Poorly healing wounds. Varicose veins.

Side effects. Sun sensitivity.

Interactions. None reported.

Overdose. None reported.

Pine Oil Pinus species, Dwarf Pine, Scotch Pine,

Stockholm Tar, Swiss Mountain Pine

Uses. Bronchial conditions. Bronchitis. Colds. Cough. Fever. Improve immune system. Nerve pain. Rheumatism. Sore throat. Inhalation. Vapors reduce bronchial secretions and local circulation. External. Antiseptic. Skin rub.

Side effects. Bronchial asthma. Kidney damage. Severe inflammation of the breathing passages. Whooping cough. External. Poisoning. Kidney damage. Brain damage. Absorbed through skin, can cause poisoning through open lesions. Skin and mucous membranes irritation.

Interactions. None reported.

Overdose. Nausea. Vomiting. Diarrhea. Dizziness. Intestinal spasms. Rash. Reddening of the face. Salivation. Shortness of breath. Sore throat. Staggering. Thirst. Twitching. Urination difficulties. Death.

Plantain Plantago

Uses. Anti-inflammatory. Antiseptic. Bites. Bruises. Burns. Cancer. Cough. Diarrhea. Dysentery. High blood pressure. Infections. Rheumatism. Snakebite. Stomachache. Warts. Weight loss.

Side effects. None reported.

Interactions. None reported. May interfere with absorption of medications.

Overdose. None reported. Plants looking similar are toxic.

Poplar Populus species, European Aspen, Quaking Aspen: contains salicylic acid

Uses. Antibacterial. Anti-inflammatory. Bladder complaints. Burns. Colds. Frostbite. Hemorrhoids. Pain. Prostate problems. Rheumatism. Spasms. Sunburn. Urinary system disorder. Wounds.

Side effects. Avoid if allergic to aspirin or Balsam of Peru. External use can cause allergic skin reactions.

Interactions. None reported. It may be reasonable to assume a blood thinning component that would affect blood thinners.

Overdose. None reported. It would be reasonable to assume an exaggeration of side effects.

Potentilla Potentilla anserina, Cinquefoil, Crampweed, Goose Tansy, Goosegrass, Moor Grass, Silverweed, Trailing Tansy, Wild Agrimony

Uses. Astringent. Diarrhea. Jaundice (liver disease). Lockjaw. Menstrual cramps. Nausea. Nervous agitation. Premenstrual syndrome (PMS). Prevent scarring from smallpox. Remove freckles. Sexual disorders. Sore throat.

Side effects. Worsen stomach problems.

Interactions. None reported.

Overdose. None reported.

Prickly Pear Opuntia

Uses. Anti-inflammatory. Antiseptic. Bites. Bruises. Burns. Diabetes. Diuretic. Insect bites. Rheumatism.
Urinary tract infections. Warts. Similar to aloe vera.

Side effects. None reported. Thorns can stick in mouth or throat.

Interactions. None reported.

Overdose. None reported.

Primrose Primula elatior, Arthritic, Butter Rose, Cowslip, Crewel, Fairy Caps, Key Flower, Mayflower, Palsywort

Uses. Asthma. Bronchitis. Cardiac insufficiency. Cough. Decongestant. Dizziness. Gout. Headache. Insomnia. Nerve pain. Skin conditions. Thin phlegm. Tremors. Whiten and smooth the skin. Whooping cough.

Side effects. Allergic reaction. Avoid if sensitive to aspirin. Uterine stimulants.

Interactions. Avoid with blood thinners.

Overdose. Diarrhea. Nausea. Stomach problems.

Psyllium Plantago ovata, Plantago ispaghula, Plantago seed, Indian Plantago, Sand Plantain, Spogel: contains fiber, muclilage

Uses. Anal fissures (cracks in the skin near the anus). Atherosclerosis. Bladder problems. Constipation. Diarrhea. Hemorrhoids. High blood pressure. High cholesterol. High triglycerides. Insect bites. Irritable bowel syndrome. Obesity. Poison ivy. Psoriasis. Skin irritations. Stings. Weight loss. Active ingredient in over-the-counter laxatives.

Side effects. Allergic reactions. Asthma. Conjunctivitis (pinkeye). Hives. Runny nose. May swell and block the esophagus or intestine. Avoid with bowel obstruction or narrowing of digestive tract. Diabetics avoid if having problems regulating blood sugar.

Interactions. May interfere with the absorption of vitamins, minerals and medications. May decrease needed dose of insulin.

Overdose. None reported.

Pumpkin Seed Cucurbita pepo

Uses. Anti-inflammatory. Antioxidant. Bowel disorders. Diabetes. Edema. Fever. Intestinal parasites. Kidney inflammation. Nausea. Prostate enlargement.
Seasickness. Urinary complaints. Wounds.

Side effects. Does not correct underlying urinary problem.

Interactions. None reported.

Overdose. None reported.

Pygeum Pygeum africanum: contains lipophilic extract, phytosterols, beta-sitosterol, Pentacyclic terpenes, ferulic esters

Uses. Anti-inflammatory. Decongestant. Edema. BPK. Urinary disorders.

Side effects. Gastrointestinal irritation. Slow acting. Delayed treatment of cancer can lead to death.

Interactions. None reported.

Overdose. None reported.

Radish Raphanus sativus

Uses. Appetite loss. Bronchitis. Colds. Cough. Digestive disorders. Fever. Headache. Improve immune system. Liver disease. Pain. Promote digestive secretions. Sore throat. Stimulate the bowels. Upper respiratory inflammation

Side effects. Biliary tract spasms with gallstones. Irritate the digestive tract.

Interactions. None reported.

Overdose. None reported.

Raspberry Rubus idaeus: contains tanning, vitamin C

Uses. Heart problems. Indigestion. Lung problems. Mouth and throat sores. Complications of pregnancy.
Stomach problems.

Side effects. None reported.

Interactions. None reported.

Overdose. None reported.

Rauwolfia Rauwolfia serpentina

Uses. Abnormal muscle tension. Antidote for poisonous snake bites. Anxiety. Constipation. Diarrhea. Diuretic (i.e. Diupres,

Hydropres). Edema. Fever. General weakness. Giddiness. High blood pressure. Insomnia. Intestinal diseases. Irregular heartbeat. Liver problems. Mental disorders. Nervousness. Rheumatism. Sedative. Slow, painful urination. Twitching. Water retention. Wounds.

Side effects. Depression. Exaggeration of depression. Fatigue. Impotence. Nasal congestion. Severe depression. Slowed reaction time. Stimulate the lining of the digestive tract. Avoid with ulcer or ulcerative colitis. Use care if driving or working with machinery.

Interactions. Avoid with monoamine oxidase inhibitor (MAOI), Nardil and Parnate. With alcohol and barbiturates increases sedation. With digitalis type drugs i.e. Lanoxin slows the heart and causes irregular beats. With quinidine products i.e. Quinaglute and Quinidex, slows the heart and causes irregular beats. With Levodopa (Sinemet) twitching and other involuntary movements. With the common flu remedies and appetite suppressants leads to sharp rise in blood pressure.

Overdose. Heavy sedation. Mental depression. Drop in blood pressure.

Redbud Cercis canadensia

Uses. Antiemetic. Diarrhea. Dysentery. Fever Leukemia. Lung congestion. Nausea. Whooping cough. Wounds.

Side effects. None reported.
Interactions. None reported.
Overdose. None reported.

Red Clover Trifolium pratense, Purple Clover, Trefoil , Wild Clover : contains isoflavone compounds, genistein, weak estrogen properties .

Uses. Acne. Boils. Bronchial spasms. Bronchitis. Cancer (breast, prostate). Cough. Diuretic. Eczema. Expectorant. Respiratory problems. Whooping cough. External. Eczema. Psoriasis.

Side effects. None reported with non-fermented red clover. Avoid fermented red clover.

Interactions. Do not take with blood thinners or aspirin.

Overdose. None reported.

Red Raspberry Rubus idaeus, contains tannins

Uses. Acute diarrhea. Common cold. Complications of pregnancy. Diarrhea. Excessive menstrual flow. Sore throat.

Side effects. Loosening of stools. Nausea.

Interactions. None reported.

Overdose. None reported. It would be reasonable assume an exaggeration of side effects.

Red Sandalwood Pterocarpus santalinus, Rubywood, Sappan

Uses. Astringent. Blood purifier. Cough. Diabetes. Diuretic. Headache. Indigestion. Skin diseases. Toothache. Vomiting.

Side effects. None reported.

Interactions. None reported.

Overdose. None reported.

Reishi Ganoderma Lucidum, Ling chih, Ling Zhi: contains sterols, coumarin, mannitol, polysaccharides, tri terpenoids, ganoderic acids

Uses. Altitude sickness. Asthma. Chemotherapy support. Cough. Decrease low density lipoproteins (LDL). Fatigue. Hepatitis support. High blood pressure. High triglycerides (hypertriglyceridemia). Insomnia. Keep blood platelets from sticking together. Weakness.

Side effects. Abdominal upset. Dizziness. Dry mouth and throat. Nose bleeds.

Interactions. Increase bleeding time. Avoid with other blood thinners.

Overdose. None reported.

Restharrow Ononis spinosa, Cammock, Ground Furze, Stayplough, Stinking Tommy, Wild Licorice

Uses. Diuretic. Gout. Kidney and bladder stones. Rheumatism. Urinary tract infections.

Side effects. Do not use with poor heart or kidney function.

Interactions. None reported.

Overdose. None reported.

Rhatany Krameria triandra, Krameria Root, Mapato

Uses. Diarrhea. Hemorrhoids. Rectal pain. Sore throat. Gargle or mouthwash. Mild inflammation of mouth, throat, or gums. External. Astringent. Frostbite. Leg throat, or gums. ulcers.

Side effects. Allergic reactions in the mucous membranes. Digestive problems.

Interactions. None reported.

Overdose. None reported.

Rhubarb Rheum palmatum, China Rhubarb, Indian Rhubarb, Russian Rhubarb, Turkey Rhubarb

Uses. Anal fissures (cracks in the skin near the anus). Bowel cleanser. Constipation. Hastens bowel movements. Hemorrhoids. Post-operative anal or rectal surgery. Soften stool.

Side effects. Cramping. Nausea. Avoid with abdominal pain, appendicitis, arthritis, colitis, Chron's, gout, inflammatory intestinal conditions or intestinal obstruction.

Interactions. Enhance action of digitalis type heart medications.

Overdose. Bone deterioration. Fluid retention. Irregular heart rhythms. Kidney problems. Laxative dependence. Leaves are toxic.

Roman Chamomile Chamaemelum nobile, Ground Apple, Whig Plant

Uses. Acne. Bloating. Boils. Cold. Eczema. General weakness. Menstrual complaints. Mild stomach and intestinal spasms. Nervousness. Sluggish bowels. Sore throat. Upset stomach. Wounds. External. Antibacterial. Antifungal. Earache. Headache. Influenza. Runny nose. Sore throat. Toothache.

Side effects. Congestion of the circulatory system. Bleeding tendency.

Interactions. Do not take with blood thinners or aspirin.

Overdose. None reported.

Rose Flower Rosa centifolia, Cabbage Rose, Damask Rose, French Rose

Uses. Astringent. Backache. Cough. Diarrhea. Dysentery. Excessive sweating. Fever. Headache. Heart trouble. Nerves. Oral inflammations. Parasites. Scurvy. Sores. Sore throat. Wounds.

Side effects. None reported.

Interactions. None reported.

Overdose. None reported.

Rose Hip Rosa canina, Briar Rose, Dog Rose, Eglantine Gall, Sweet Briar, Wild Brier, Witches' Brier

Uses. Gout. Improve immune system. Kidney disease. Laxative effect. Rheumatism. Sciatica (nerve pain in the lower back and thigh). Source of vitamin C. Urinary tract infections. Water retention.

Side effects. None reported.

Interactions. None reported.

Overdose. None reported.

Rosemary Rosmarinus officinalis, Compass-weed, Polar Plant

Uses. Appetite loss. Blood pressure. Decrease spasms in the gallbladder and upper intestine. Female sexual disorders. Improve blood flow to heart. Improves memory. Liver and gallbladder problems. Rheumatism. Strengthen heart muscle action. External. Eczema. Improves circulation. Poorly healing wounds.

Side effects. Contact skin reactions.

Interactions. None reported.

Overdose. None reported. One theory states could cause coma, spasm, vomiting, digestive tract inflammation, uterine bleeding, abortion, kidney irritation, swelling in the lungs, and death.

Rue Ruta graveolens, Herb-of-Grace

Uses. Contraceptive. Cramps. Diarrhea. Earache. Fever. Hepatitis. Indigestion. Intestinal worms. Menstrual disorders (PMS). Skin inflammation. Sore throat. Sprains. Strains. Toothache.

Side effects. Sun sensitivity.

Interactions. None reported.

Overdose. Delirium. Depression. Dizziness. Fainting. Liver and kidney damage. Sleep disorders. Spasm. Stomach pain. Tremor. Vomiting. Death.

Rupturewort Herniaria glabra, Flax Weed, Herniary

Uses. Gout. Hernias. Increase urination. Kidney stones. Nerve inflammation. Relieve spasms. Respiratory disorders. Rheumatism. Urinary tract infections.

Side effects. None reported.

Interactions. None reported.

Overdose. None reported.

Saffron Crocus Sativus

Uses. Control bleeding. Depression. Difficult labor. Digestive problems. Enhances production of gastric juices. Inflammation. Menstrual disorders. Throat diseases. Vomiting.

Side effects. Abortion.

Interactions. None reported. May increase effects of blood thinners.

Overdose. Bleeding from the lips and eyelids. Bleeding from uterus. Blood in the urine. Bloody diarrhea. Dizziness. Intestinal cramping. Nose bleeds. Paralysis. Poisoning. Red or purple blotches. Stupor. Vomiting. Yellowing of the skin. Death.

Sage Salvia Officinalis

Uses. Appetite loss. Bloating. Blood in phlegm. Blood in the urine. Diarrhea. Excessive flow of breast milk. Excessive perspiration. Fluid in the abdomen. Gargle for bleeding gums. Gargle for sore throats. Insect bites. Intestinal inflammation. Sexually transmitted disease. Sore throat. Type II non-insulin dependent diabetes. External. Astringent. Antibacterial. Antifungal. Antiviral. Mild injuries. Hemorrhoids. Reduces perspiration. Skin inflammation.

Side effects. Increase seizures in people with epilepsy. Avoid with heart disorders.

Interactions. None reported.

Overdose. Convulsions. Dizziness. Feeling of warmth. Rapid heartbeat.

Sandalwood Santalum album, Sanderswood, White Saunders: contain alpha- and beta-santalol
Uses. Abdominal pain. Abnormal thirst. Acne. Astringent. Bronchitis. Burning sensation. Colds. Cough. Difficult swallowing. Disinfectant. Diuretic. Dysentery. Excessive sex drive. Expectorant. Fever. Fragrance. Gonorrhea. Headache. Heatstroke. Improve immune system. Liver and gallbladder problems. Sedation. Skin diseases. Sore throat. Stomach pain. Sunstroke. Urinary tract infections. Urinary problems. Vomiting. Essential oil has medicinal effects.
Side effects. Blood in urine. Intestinal problems. Itchy skin. Queasiness. Skin irritation. Avoid with kidney disease. May cause kidney damage.
Interactions. None reported.
Overdose. None reported. It would be reasonable to assume an exaggeration of side effects.

Sanicle Sanicula europaea, Poolroot
Uses. Astringent. Bronchitis. Cough. Expectorant. Nervous problems.
Side effects. None reported.
Interactions. None reported.
Overdose. None reported.

Sarsaparilla Smilax spp: contains steroidal saponins, sarsasapogenin, phytosterols, beta-sitosterol
Uses. Anti- inflammatory. Cancer. Eczema. Epilepsy.

Leprosy. Liver-protecting effects. Malignant ulcers. Psoriasis. Rheumatism. Rheumatoid arthritis. Skin diseases. Syphilis. Tuberculosis. Urinary tract infections.

Side effects. Kidney damage. Nausea. Stomach complaints. Avoid long term use.

Interactions. Increase effects of bismuth. Increase effects of digitalis type medications.

Overdose. Diarrhea. Fluid loss. Shock.

Savin Tops Juniperus sabina

Uses. Warts. Oil kills the viruses that cause warts.

Side effects. For external use only. Contact with normal skin causes blistering or death of skin. Absorption through skin may cause internal poisoning.

Interactions. None reported.

Overdose. Not for internal use. Six drops of the oils can be life-threatening. Queasiness. Irregular heartbeat. Spasms. Kidney damage. Bloody urine. Paralysis. Coma. Death.

Saw Palmetto Serenoa repens, Sabal serrulata: Contains lipophilic (fat-soluble) extract, sterols, fatty acids, caproic, lauric, palmitic

Uses. Enlarged prostate. Promote normal urination. Reduce absorption of male hormones in the prostate gland. Reduce inflammation and swelling of prostate. Relieve bladder obstruction.

Side effects. Stomach complaints. Will not shrink prostate. Does not affect measuring of prostate-specific antigen (PSA).

Interactions. May have additive effects with other hormone therapies, i.e. birth control pills or estrogen replacement. Do not take with iron.

Overdose. None reported

Schisandra Schisandra chinensis, Wu-wei-zi: contains essential oils, numerous acids, lignans, Schizandrin, deoxyschizandrin, gomisins, pregomisin

Uses. Allergic skin reactions. Chemotherapy support. Common cold. Coughs. Exhaustion. Fatigue. Hepatitis support. Insomnia. Kidney tonic. Liver support. Lung astringent. Night sweats. Sore throat. Stress. Thirst. Wheezing.

Side effects. Abdominal upset. Decreased appetite. Heartburn. Skin rash.

Interactions. None reported.

Overdose. Difficulty breathing. Insomnia. Restlessness.

Scopola Scopolia carniolica, Belladonna Scopola, Japanese Belladonna

Uses. Improve conduction of electrical impulses in the heart. Liver and gallbladder problems. Relieve muscular tremors and rigidity. Relieve spasms in the digestive system, bile ducts and urinary tract. speed heart rate. Primary ingredient of prescription hyoscyamine as in Cytospaz, Donnatal, Levsin, and Urised.

Side effects. Worsen rapid heartbeat. Avoid with glaucoma. Avoid with narrowing of digestive tract or enlarged colon. Avoid with prostate tumor.

Interactions. Increase effect of some medications. Avoid with Amantadine (Symmetrel), Quinidine (Quinaglute , Quinidex) , Tri cyclic antidepressant medications i.e. Elavil, Pamelor, and Tofranil .

Overdose. Compulsive speech. Decreased perspiration. Delirium. Difficulty focusing. Dilated pupils. Dry mouth. Exhaustion. Hallucinations. Increased body heat. Manic episodes. Rapid heartbeat. Restlessness. Severe constipation. Skin reddening. Sleep. Urination problems.

Scullcap Scutellaria lateriflora, Blue Pimpernel, Helmet Flower, Hoodwort, Mad-dog Weed, Madweed, Quaker Bonnet, Member of the mint family: contains scutellaria
Uses. Anti-inflammatory. Antispasmodic. Anxiety. Epilepsy. Insomnia. Nervous tension. Nerve pain. Reduce inflammation. Sedative. Chinese scullcap: Allergies. Antibacterial. Antiseptic. Antiviral. Depression. Diarrhea. High blood pressure. Hysteria. Neuralgia.
Protective effects on the liver.
Side effects. Jitters. Restlessness.
Interactions. None reported.
Overdose. None reported.

Selenicereus Grandiflorus, Selenicereus grandiflorus, Night-blooming Cereus, Sweet -scented Cactus
Uses. Angina. Digitalis-like effects. Heart conditions. Heavy or painful menstrual periods.
Hemorrhages. Improves heart action. Opens blood vessels. Shortness of breath. Spasmodic pain. Spitting up blood.
Stimulates movement governing nerves in the spinal cord. External. Urinary tract infections. Water retention.
Anti-inflammatory effect on the skin. Rheumatism.
Side effects. Burning of the mouth. Diarrhea. Queasiness. Vomiting. External. Itching. Pustules on the skin.
Interactions. None reported.
Overdose. None reported. It would be reasonable to assume an exaggeration of side effects.

Seneca Snakeroot, Polygala senega, Milkwort, Mountain Flax, Rattlesnake Root
Uses. Bronchitis. Cough. Decongestant. Loosen phlegm.
Side effects. Irritation of digestive tract.
Interactions. None reported.
Overdose Diarrhea. Nausea. Queasiness. Stomach complaints.

Senna Cassia senna, Cassia angustifolia : contains anthraquinone glycosides, sennosides, rhein-anthrone.
Uses. Internal. Bronchitis. Cathartic. Constipation. Dysentery. Fever. Indigestion. Laxative. Seizures.
Ingredient in Senokot, Fletcher's Castoria, and Ex-Lax Gentle Nature).
External. Acne. Ringworm. Skin diseases.
Side effects. Abdominal cramps. Blood in urine. Bone loss. Dehydration. Diarrhea. Kidney disorders. Laxative dependence. Muscle weakness. Water retention. Loss of fluids. Low potassium levels. Negative effects on the heart and muscles. Avoid with intestinal blockage, appendicitis, ulcerative colitis or Crohn's disease.
Interactions. Increase the effect of digitalis like heart medications i.e. digoxin (Lanoxin). Interfere with drugs that regulate heartbeat.
Overdose. None reported. It would be reasonable to assume an exaggeration of side effects.

Shepherd's Purse Capsella bursa pastoris, Blindweed, Case-weed, Cocowort, Lady's Purse, Mother's Heart, Pepper-and-Salt, Pick-Pocket, St. James Wort
Uses. Astringent. Blood pressure. Burns. Cystitis. Diarrhea. Diuretic. Headache. Improve force and speed of heartbeat. Increase uterine contractions. Irregular heartbeat. Irregular or excessive menstrual bleeding. Malaria. Nose bleeds. Parasites. Poison

Premenstrual syndrome (PMS). Quinine substitute. Superficial bleeding from skin injuries. Swelling and urinary tract infections. Weak heart. Wounds.

Side effects. None reported.
Interactions. None reported.
Overdose. None reported.

Shiitake Lentinan edodes, Hua gu: contains proteins, fats, carbohydrates, soluble fiber, vitamins, minerals, polysaccharide, lentinan, LEM (Lentinan edodes mycelium extract), lignangs, cortinelin.

Uses. Antibacterial. Chemotherapy support. Cholesterol-lowering properties. Colds. Hepatitis support. HIV support. Increase energy. Poor circulation. Recurrent stomach cancer. Worms.

Side effects. Abdominal bloating. Temporary diarrhea.
Interactions. If combined with other herbs, it may be necessary to lower the dose. Do not take with blood thinners or aspirin.
Overdose. None reported. It would be reasonable to assume an exaggeration of side effects.

Siberian Ginseng Eleutherococcus senticosus
Uses. Improve immune system. Increase energy and Concentration. Increase levels of infection-fighting blood cells. Relieve fatigue.

Side effects. Avoid with high blood pressure.
Interactions. Increase effects of caffeine and other stimulants. Do not combine with antipsychotic drugs, steroids or hormones. Do not take with diabetic medications. Do not take with blood thinners or aspirin. Do not take with lanoxin.

Overdose. Anxiety. Headaches. High blood pressure. Insomnia. Irritability. Melancholy Palpitations. Pericardial pain.

Slippery Elm Ulmus rubra, Ulmus fulva, American Elm, Indian Elm, Moose Elm, Red Elm, Rock Elm, Sweet Elm, Winged Elm: contains mucilage
Uses. Common cold. Cough. Crohn's disease. Diarrhea. Gastritis. Skin conditions. Sore throat.
Side effects. None reported.
Interactions. None reported. May interfere with the absorption of vitamins, minerals and medications.
Overdose. None reported.

Soapwort Saponaria officinal is, Bouncing Bet Bruisewort, Crow Soap, Dog Cloves, Fuller's Herb, Latherwort, Old Maids' Pink, Soap Root, Sweet Betty, Wild Sweet William
Uses. Antibacterial. Asthma. Bronchitis. Colds. Constipation. Cough. Eczema. Expectorant action. Gout.
Loosens phlegm. Rheumatism. Venereal disease. External. Acne. Boils. Dandruff. Eczema. Persistent skin problems. Poison oak. Psoriasis.
Side effects Irritate stomach. Irritate mucous membranes.
Interactions. None reported.
Overdose. Vomiting.

Soy Lecithin Lecithinum ex soja, genistein
Uses. Appetite loss. Chest fullness. Feeling of pressure in the area of the liver. Fevers. Fidgeting. Headache. High cholesterol. Liver disease. Menopausal symptoms. Reduce the risk of estrogen-dependent tumors.

Side effects. Digestive upsets. Stomach pain. Loose stools. Diarrhea.

Interactions. None reported.

Overdose. None reported.

Spearmint Mentha spicata, Curled Mint, Fish Mint, Garden Mint, Green Mint, Lamb Mint, Mackerel Mint, Our Lady's Mint, Sage of Bethlehem, Spire Mint

Uses. Bath additive. Bee and wasp stings. Gargle. Gas. Indigestion. Flavoring agent in toothpaste, chewing gum, and certain food preparations. Washing agent.

Side effects. Allergic reaction.

Interactions. None reported.

Overdose. None reported.

Spinach Spinacia oleracea

Uses. Anemia. Appetite loss. Energizing effects. Indigestion. Relieve fatigue. Speed recovery from illnesses.

Side effects. High in nitrates. May aggravate gout.

Interactions. None reported.

Overdose. None reported.

Squill Drimia oleracea

Uses. Cough. High blood pressure. Increase strength of heart contractions. Irregular heartbeat. Pneumonia. Poor kidneys. Rheumatism. Slows heartbeat. Vein problems. Weak heart.

Side effects. Diarrhea. Digestive spasms. Headache. Irregular pulse. Loss of appetite. Vomiting. Skin contact causes skin inflammation.

Interactions. Heart irregularities increases when combined with: Asthma medications, i.e. Alupent, Proventil, and theophylline

Theo-Dur. Heart medications i.e. Inocor, Primacor, Quinidine, Quinaglute, Quinidex. Water pills (diuretics). Laxatives. Steroid drugs i.e. prednisone.

Overdose. Confusion. Depression. Hallucinations. Psychosis. Serious heartbeat irregularities. Stupor. Vision disorders. Cardiac arrest. Asphyxiation.

St. Johns Wort Hypericum perforatum, Amber, Goatweed, Hardhay, Klamath Weed, Tipton Weed: contains hypericin, pseudohypericin, xanthones, flavonoids

Uses. AIDS. Antiviral. Anxiety. Asthma. Bed-wetting. Bronchitis. Bruises. Burns. Depression. Diarrhea. Gallbladder disorders. Gastritis. Gout. Hemorrhoids. Kidney disorders. Lung disorders. Muscle pain. Poisonous reptile bites. Recurrent ear infections. Rheumatism. Sciatica. Skin inflammation. Sleep disturbances. Vitiligo. Wounds.

Side effects. Bloating. Cataracts hypersensitivity. Constipation. Nerve hypersensitivity. Sun sensitivity.

Interactions. Avoid foods like red wine, cheese, yeast, and pickled herring. Do not use with MAO inhibitors or Parkinson's medications, such as furazolidone (Furoxone), isocarboxazid (Marplan), procarbazine (Matulane) , selegiline (Eldepryl) , moclobemide (Manerex) , phenelzine (Nardil) or Parnate . Interactions include a sudden, dangerous surge in blood pressure. Prolong anesthesia effects. Do not take with dextromethorphan (in cough medicines). Do not take with SSRIs or antidepressants. Do not take with Tetracycline. Do not take with Thorazine. Do not take with iron. Do not take with heart medications. Do not take with alcohol, barbiturates or Valium type medications. Do not take with theophylline. Do not take with birth control pills. Do not take with cholesterol medications. Do not take with medications commonly used in the treatment of HIV or AIDS. Do not take with immune suppressing medications.

Overdose. None reported.

Star Anise Illicium verum, Aniseed Stars, Badiana, Chinese Anise

Uses. Appetite loss. Arthritis. Bronchitis. Cough. Facial paralysis. Indigestion. Intestinal cramps. Loosen phlegm. Promote digestion. Sweeten breath.

Side effects. Sensitivity to herb. Do not confuse with the poisonous Japanese star anise.

Interactions. None reported.

Overdose. None reported.

Stinging Nettle Urtica dioica, Dwarf Nettle, Greater Nettle, Nettle Wort

Uses. Kidney and bladder stones. Prostate enlargement. Relieves symptoms of frequent urination and weak urinary flow. Rheumatism. Urinary tract infections. Diuretic. "Diabetic teas. Itching. Spleen conditions. External. Oily hair. Dandruff.

Side effects. Mild stomach and intestinal problems. Skin reactions. Swelling. Avoid with a heart or kidney condition.

Interactions. None reported.

Overdose. None reported. It would be reasonable to assume an exaggeration of side effects.

Strawberry Fragaria vesca

Uses. Astringent. Diarrhea. Digestive problems. Diuretic. Gout. Kidney stones. Liver disease. Rash.
Respiratory tract inflammation. Rheumatism. Tension. Water retention.

Side effects. Allergic reaction.
Interactions. None reported.
Overdose. None reported.

Sundew Drosera rotundifolia, Dew Plant, Lustwort, Red
Rot, Youthwort
    Uses. Arteriosclerosis. Asthma. Bronchial spasms. Bronchitis.
Cough. Decongestant. Warts.
    Side effects. None reported.
    Interactions. None reported.
    Overdose. None reported.

Sunflower Helianthus
    Uses. Arthritis. Boils. Diabetes. Diarrhea. Diuretic.
Expectorant. Fever. Malaria. Snakebite. Spider bites.
    Side effects. Allergic reactions.
    Interactions. None reported.
    Overdose. None reported.

Sweet Clover Melilotus official is, Hart's Tree, Hay
Flowers, King's Clover, Melilot, Sweet Lucerne, Wild
Laburnum: contains coumarin
    Uses. Anti-inflammatory. Blood clots. Bruises. Diuretic.
Headache. Hemorrhage. Hemorrhoids. Itching. Leg heaviness. Leg
pain. Leg swelling. Lymph system congestion. Night cramps. Poor
circulation. Vein inflammation. External. Speed healing of bruises.
    Side effects Headache. Stupor. Temporary liver damage.
    Interactions. Avoid with blood thinners.
    Overdose. None reported. It would be reasonable to assume
an exaggeration of side effects.

Sweet Violet Sweet Violet Viola odorata, Garden Violet
   Uses. Antimicrobial. Asthma. Bronchitis. Calming effect.
Colds. Cough. Fever. Headaches. Insomnia. Loosen phlegm. Migraine.
Promote urination. Promote vomiting.
Quell anger. Rheumatism. Skin diseases. Sore throat. Stress.
   Side effects. None reported.
   Interactions. None reported.
   Overdose. None reported.

   Tangerine Peel Citrus reticulata, Mandarin Orange
Peel
   Uses. Bloating. Gas. Hernia. Indigestion. Loose stools. Nausea.
Pain in the breast and side. Vomiting. With pinellia root used to
loosen phlegm and relieve chest congestion.
   Side effects. Avoid with a dry cough, an excessively red
tongue, or if spitting up blood.
   Interactions. None reported.
   Overdose. None reported.

   Tea Tree Melaleuca alternifolia: contains terpenoids, terpinen
and cineole
   Uses. Acne. Antibacterial. Antifungal. Athletes foot. Cuts.
Disinfectant. Skin infections. Vaginitis. Yeast infections.
   Side effects. None reported.
   Interactions. None reported.
   Overdose. None reported.

   Thyme Thymus vulgaris: contains Thymol
   Uses. Antibacterial. Bronchial spasms. Bronchitis. Cough.
Deodorant skin rub. Digestive aid. Diuretic. Expectorant. Gas.

Inflammation of upper respiratory tract. Urinary disinfectant. Whooping cough. Worms.

Side effects. Irritate mucous membranes.

Interactions. None reported.

Overdose. None reported.

Tormentil Potentilla erecta, Bloodroot, English Sarsaparilla, Ewe Daisy, Sept foil, Shepherd's Knot

Uses. Astringent. Diarrhea. Inflammation of stomach and intestines. Sore throat.

Side effects. Digestive disorders. Vomiting.

Interactions. None reported.

Overdose. None reported.

Tree of Heaven Ailanthus altissima, Ailanto, Chinese Sumac, Vernis de Japon

Uses. Asthma. Astringent. Calm spasms. Cramps. Diarrhea. Epilepsy. Fast heart rate. Fever. Gonorrhea. Malaria. Painful menstruation. Vaginal discharges. Worm infestation.

Side effects. Diarrhea. Dizziness. Headache. Nausea. Tingling in the arms and legs.

Interactions. None reported.

Overdose. Fatal poisonings in animals.

True Unicorn Aletris farinosa, Ague Grass, Aloe-root, Bettie Grass, Black-root, Colic Root, Crow Corn, Devil's Bit, Star Root, Starwort

Uses. Blood disorders. Bronchitis. Digestive problems. Gas. Indigestion. Loss of appetite. Menstrual problems. Nervous stomach. Poor digestion. Prevent threatened miscarriage. Symptoms of prolapsed uterus.

Side effects. Fresh root. Vomiting.
Interactions. None reported.
Overdose. None reported.

Tumeric Curcuma longa, Curcuma domestica: contains curcumin
Uses. Antibacterial. Antioxidant. Anti-tumor. Appetite loss. Atherosclerosis. Bloating. Bronchitis. Bruises. Bursitis. Cancer prevention. Chest infections. Colds. Constipation. Coughs. Cramps. Diarrhea. Festering eye infection. Fever. Gas. Headaches. Increase milk production. Indigestion. Infected wounds. Inflamed skin. Inflammation. Inflammation in the mouth. Intestinal infections. Kidney and bladder inflammation. Leech bites. Leprosy. Liver and gallbladder problems. Missed menstrual periods. Poor vision. Protects the liver from toxic compounds. Reduce platelets clumping. Rheumatoid arthritis. Skin diseases. Stomach pain. Swelling. Worms.
Side effects. Stomach problems. Avoid with gallstones.
Interactions. None reported. May increase bleeding. Avoid with blood thinners.
Overdose. Stomach problems.

Usnea Beard Moss, Old Man's Beard, Tree Moss
Uses. Baldness. Cough. Disinfectant. Eye irritation. Headache. Malaria. Problems in the uterus. Respiratory infections. Sore throat. Sunstroke. Vaginal discharge.
Side effects. None reported.
Interactions. None reported.
Overdose. None reported. May be poisonous.

Uva Ursi Arctostaphylos uva-ursi, bearberry: contains glycoside arbutin, Hydroquinone

Uses. Antimicrobial. Astringent. Infections. Urinary tract infections in alkaline urine. Weight-loss aid.

Side effects. Nausea.

Interactions. Increase the anti-inflammatory effect of non-steroidal medications (NSAIDS). Avoid with acidic agents, i.e. fruit juice or Vitamin C.

Overdose. None reported.

Uzara Xysmalobium undulatum: contains uzarone

Uses. Diarrhea. Dysentery. Steady heartbeat. Strengthen heart contractions.

Side effects. None reported.

Interactions. Avoid with heart medications, especially digitalis- type medications i.e. digoxin, Lanoxin).

Overdose. None reported.

Valerian Valeriana officinal is, All-heal, Amantilla, Capon's Tail, Heliotrope, Setwall, Vandal Root

Uses. Anxiety. Colic. Digestive problems. Epilepsy. Excitability. Fainting. Headache. Hysteria. Insomnia. Lack of concentration. Liver problems. Menopause. Mental strain. Nausea. Nerve pain. Nervous conditions. Premenstrual syndrome. Relaxes muscles. Sedative. Stomach cramps. Stress. Symptoms of pregnancy. Urinary tract disorders. Uterine spasms.

Side effects. Allergic reaction. Digestive problems. Headache. Heart problems. Pupil dilation. Restlessness. Sleeplessness. Avoid with a large skin injury or open lesions. Avoid with heart problems or severe muscle tens ion.

Interactions. Interferes with anti-anxiety medications, hypnotics, analgesics, and anti-epileptics. Increases the effects of kava, passionflower, lemon balm, hops, poppy and skullcap. Will enhance and prolong barbiturate effect. Avoid with alcohol. Do not take with Flagyl.

Overdose. None reported.

Verbena Verbena officinal is, Herb of Grace, Juno's Tears, Pigeon's Grass, Simpler's Joy, Vervain

Uses. Abdominal distention. Anti-cancer agent. Anti-inflammatory. Antimicrobial. Antiviral. Asthma.
Bronchitis. Cough. Cramps. Digestive disorders. Fatigue. Gout. Improve immune system. Kidney stones. Kidney and urinary tract complications. Liver and gallbladder diseases. Malaria. Menopause. Menstrual problems.
Nervous disorders. Pain. Rheumatism. Sore throat.
Stimulate production of breast milk. Water retention. External. Arthritis. Bruises. Dislocations. Itching.
Pain of minor burns.

Side effects. None reported.

Interactions. None reported.

Overdose. Vomiting.

Veronica Veronica officinal is, Speedwell

Uses. Boils. Chronic skin conditions. Cough. Diarrhea. Fever Gargle. Heal ulcers. Hepatitis.
Indigestion. Kidney problems. Liver disorders. Nervous agitation. Prevent ulcers. Respiratory ailments. Rheumatism. Sore throat. "Tired blood." Urinary tract infections. External. Relieve itching. Speed wound healing. "Sweating of the feet."

Side effects. None reported.

Interactions. None reported.

Overdose. None reported.

Violet Viola

Uses. Bites. Blood tonic. Bronchitis. Constipation. Cough. Diaper rash. Diarrhea. Eczema. Eyewash. Fever. Headache. Insomnia. Lung congestion. Sores. Varicose veins.

Side effects. Vomiting.

Interactions. None reported.

Overdose. None reported. It would be reasonable to assume an exaggeration of side effects.

Vitex Agnus-castus, Chaste tree, Monk's pepper

Uses. Assist with the passing of the afterbirth. Fibrocystic breast disease. Hemorrhage following childbirth. Increases progesterone production. Infertility (female). Menopause. Menorrhagia (heavy menstruation). Menstrual difficulties (secondary amenorrhea). Pre-menstrual syndrome. Regulate menstrual cycle. Stimulate production of breast milk. Suppress libido and inspire chastity. External. Sitz baths for diseases of uterus.

Side effects. Minor gastrointestinal upset. Mild itchy skin rash.

Interactions. May interfere with Reglan, Haldol, Prolixin, and Thorazine. Do not take with estrogen.

Overdose. None reported. It would be reasonable to assume an exaggeration of side effects.

Walnut

Uses. Antifungal. Astringent. Cholesterol. Eczema. Excessive perspiration. Herpes. Inflammation of the digestive tract. Intestinal worms. Skin inflammation. Syphilis. Tuberculosis.

Side effects. None reported.

Interactions. None reported.

Overdose. None reported.

Watercress Nasturtium officinale, Indian Cress: contains mustard oil

Uses. Arthritis. Bactericidal. Bronchitis. Compresses. Constipation. Cough. Diuretic. General tonic. Improve digestion. Liver disorders. Nervous conditions. Source of Vitamin C. Stimulate appetite.

Side effects. Irritation of the stomach and intestines.

Interactions. None reported.

Overdose. None reported. It would be reasonable to assume an exaggeration of side effects.

White Nettle Lamium album, Archangel, Bee Nettle, White Deadnettle

Uses. Astringent. Bronchitis. Cough. Digestive disorders. Expectorant. Female sexual disorders. Loosen phlegm. Menopausal complaints. Skin inflammation. Sore throat. Urinary problems.

Side effects. None reported.

Interactions. None reported.

Overdose. None reported.

White willow Salix alba, European Willow, Salicin Willow: contains glycoside salicin, salicylic acid

Uses. Bursitis. Fever. Headache (tension). Jaundice. Osteoarthritis. Pain. Rheumatoid arthritis.

Side effects. Diarrhea. Gastrointestinal irritation. Nausea.

Interactions. Avoid if allergic or cannot take aspirin or anti-inflammatories.

Overdose. None reported.

Wild Cherry Prunus serotina, Choke Cherry, Rum Cherry, Virginian Prune: contains cyanogenic glycosides, prunasin

Uses. Bronchitis. Cough. Diarrhea. Indigestion. Lung problems. Nervous stomach. Pain relief.

Side effects. None reported.

Interactions. None reported.

Overdose. None reported. Technically might prove fatal.

Wild Thyme Thymus serpyllum, Mother of Thyme, Shepherd's Thyme

Uses. Anti-spasmodic. Asthma. Bactericidal. Bronchitis. Cough. Diarrhea. Gas. Headaches. Itching. Kidney and bladder disorders. Loosen phlegm. Nightmares. Rheumatism. Sprains. Stimulate digestion. Stimulates secretions. Toothache. Uterine disorders. Vomiting. Whooping cough.

Side effects. None reported.

Interactions. None reported.

Overdose. None reported.

Wild Yam Dioscorea villosa, China Root, Colic Root, Devil 's Bones, Rheumatism Root, Yuma: contains saponins, diosgenin (that may change into cortisone) , estrogens, progesterone-like compounds .

Uses. Abdominal cramps. Anti-inflammatory. Antioxidant. Expectorant. Gallbladder problems. High cholesterol. High triglycerides (hypertriglyceridemia). Lower blood sugar. Menopause. Morning sickness. Muscle pain or spasms. Nerve pain. Painful menstruation. Rheumatism. Stomach upset.

Side effects. Nausea.

Interactions. None reported.

Overdose. None reported.

Wintergreen Gaultheria procumbens, Boxberry, Canada Tea, Checkerberry, Deerberry, Ground Berry, Hillberry, Mountain Tea, Partridge Berry, Spiceberry, Teaberry, Wax Cluster

Uses. Rheumatism. External. Pain of rheumatoid arthritis. Muscle, joint, or nerve pain. Stomach pain. Back pain. Inflammation. Painful menstruation. Antiseptic. Asthma. In remedies as Bengay an Arthricare...

Side effects. Contact allergies.

Interactions. None reported.

Overdose. Severe stomach and kidney irritation. Central nervous system problems. Fluid build-up in the lungs. Collapse. Death.

Witch Hazel Hamamelis virginiana, Snapping Hazelnut, Spotted Alder, Tobacco Wood, Winterbloom: contains tannins and volatile oils

Uses. Anti-inflammatory. Astringent. Beneficial effect on veins. Burns. Colitis. Coughing up blood. Diarrhea. Eczema. Hemorrhoids. Insect bites. Menstrual complaints. Skin ulcers. Varicose veins. Vomiting. Wound healing. External. Compress for painful swellings. Stops bleeding.

Side effects. Minor skin irritation. Do not take internally. If taken internally, can cause digestive problems. Risk of liver damage.

Interactions. None reported.

Overdose. None reported. It would be reasonable to assume an exaggeration of side effects.

Woodruff Woodruff Galium odorata: contains coumarin

Uses. Anti-inflammatory. Edginess. Insomnia. Irregular heartbeat. Menstrual disorders. Relieve swelling and spasms. Urinary tract infections. Water retention.
Side effects. Liver damage.
Interactions. Can increase effects of blood thinners.
Overdose. Headache. Disorientation. Liver damage.

Yarrow Achillea millefolium, Bloodwort, Devil ' s Nettle, Milfoil, Sanguinary, Staunchweed
Uses. Appetite loss. Astringent. Gallbladder disorders. Headache. Improve bile flow. Indigestion. Liver disorders. Menstrual problems. Pelvic cramps. Relieve muscle spasms in the intestines. Soothe the digestive system. External. Astringent. Antibacterial. Bruises. Burns. Relieve skin inflammation. Stop bleeding.
Side effects. Allergic reaction. Sun sensitivity.
Interaction. None reported.
Overdose. Uterine stimulant. Avoid during pregnancy.

Yellow Dock Rumex crispus, Curled Dock
Uses. Blood cleanser. Constipation. Cough. Improve immune system. Itching. Liver and gallbladder problems. Pain. Respiratory tract disorders. Skin inflammation.
Side effects. Vomiting.
Interactions. None reported.
Overdose. Poisoning for fresh yellow dock.

Yohimbe Pausinystalia yohimbe, Corynanthe yohimbe: contains yohimbine, quebrachine, aphrodine, corynine
Uses. Aphrodisiac. Coughs. Depression. Dilates blood vessels. Dilates pupils. Fevers. Heart disease. Inhibits monamine oxidase. Local anesthetic. Leprosy. Male impotence/ infertility.

Side effects. Aggravate heart disease, liver disease, kidney disease or peptic ulcers. Agitation. Anxiety. Dizziness. Fast heartbeat, Hallucinations. Headache. High blood pressure. Insomnia. Nausea. Sleeplessness. Tremors. Vomiting. Larger doses. Chills. Loss of muscle function. Tremors. Vertigo.

Interactions. Severe high blood pressure if taken with cheese, red wine, liver, yeast containing foods, i.e. yogurt. Do not take with anti-depressants. Do not take with blood pressure medications.

Overdose. Salivation. Dilated pupils. Loss of control of the bowels. Low blood pressure. Irregular heartbeat. Heart failure. Death.

Yucca Yucca schidigera: contains saponins

Uses. Bleeding. Fights dandruff. Foaming agent in root beer. Hair loss. Joint inflammations. Osteoarthritis. Poultices for skin sores and sprains. Promote normal formation of cartilage. Rheumatoid arthritis. Shampoo.

Side effects. Loose stools. In theory, may cause the red blood cells to burst.

Interactions. None reported.

Overdose. None reported.

Zedoary Curcuma zedoaria

Uses. Bloating. Combat digestive spasms. Cramps. Digestive problems. Gas. Heartburn. Heavy menstrual flow. Improve bile flow. Indigestion. Nausea. Nervous diseases. Stimulate production of digestive juices. Stomach pain.

Side effects. None reported.

Interactions. None reported.

Overdose. None reported.

Resources

American Society of Anesthesiologists. Possible Side effects and Drug Interactions herb2. Available: http://www.asahq.org/profinfo/herb/list.

Bell, Howard. Drs. Guide to BPH on the Web. Available: www.pslgroup.com/enlargprost.htm

Caufield, C. (1984). In the Rainforest: Report from a Strange, Beautiful, Imperiled World. Chicago, IL: University of Chicago Press.

Debaggio, T., and Belsinger, S. (1996). Basil, an Herb Lover's Guide. Loveland, CO: Interweave Press.

HealthGate Data Corp. (1999). Complete Guide to vitamins, Minerals & Supplements. Available: http://www.healthgate.com

Heatherley, A. (1998). Healing Plants: A medicinal guide to native North American plants and herbs. New York: The Lyons Press.

Integrative Medicine Nursing Consult. Reference to Botanical Medicines 1999. Newton Mass.: Integrative Medicine Communications.

Kuhn, M. (2002). Herbal drug remedies: Drug-herb interactions. Critical Care Nurse 22, 2. P22. Aliseo Viejo, Ca.: Innovation

Lininger, S., Wright, J., Austin, S., Brown, D., and Gaby, A. (1998) The Natural Pharmacy. Virtual Health, LLC. Rocklin, Ca: Prima Publishing

Loecher, B. (2000). Brave New Botanicals. Prevention Guide Healing Herbs January 21, 2000. Emmaus Pa:

McVicar, Jekka. (1994). Herbs for the home. New York: Viking Studio Books.

Medical Economics Company. (1999). PDR for Herbal Medicines. First edition. Montvale, New Jersey: Medical Economics Company.

Medical Economics Company, Inc. (1999). Alternative medicine: Herbal Remedies. Available: Yahoo! Inc. Yahoo! Health
Murray, M. (1995). The Healing Power of Herbs. 2nd ed. Rocklin, CA.: Prima Publishing

NIH Office of Dietary Supplements. Available: http://odp.od.nih.gov/ods/question.html

Prevention Guide (2000). Healing Herbs July 21, 2000. Emmaus Pa: Prevention

Prevention Guide (2000). Herbs for Health. Emmaus, Pa.: Prevention

Raintree Nutrition, Inc. Welcome to wealth of the Rainforest: Pharmacy to the World. Available: http://www.rain-tree.com

Reader's Digest (1986). Magic and Medicine of Plants. New York: Reader's Digest Association

Schar, D. (2000). Gifts of the Magi. Prevention Guide Healing Herbs January 21, 2000. Emmaus Pa:

Tien, R. and Schellekens, E. (1999). The Guide to Surname. Amsterdam: Brasa Publishers.

Tyler, V. The Honest Herbalist: A Sensible Guide to the Use of Herbs and Related Remedies. Binghamton, NY: Pharmaceutical

Muscle & Fitness. (1999). Power Plants: 49 Herbs to build muscle, burn fat & boost energy. New York: Weider Publications.

ABOUT THE AUTHOR

A registered nurse working full time in the emergency room, Kay A Fox has her master's degree in nursing and is a certified emergency nurse. Ms. Fox' s continued education includes the integrative therapies of hypnosis, healing, acupressure/reflexology, and the use of herbs. She believes all people have the right to the best care available. That means working as a team with the whole person, body, mind and spirit. Members of the team need information to help with decision-making. To that end she has produced A BASIC GUIDE TO HERBS to provide nurses, doctors and consumers of health care with a quick and easy guide to one of the fastest growing arenas of integrative medicine, herbal therapy.

www.ingramcontent.com/pod-product-compliance
Lightning Source LLC
Chambersburg PA
CBHW070840300326
41935CB00038B/1160